30 DAY WHOLE FOOD CHALLENGE:

Over 100 Delicious Whole Food Recipes to Lose Weight and Stay Fit

by

Amanda Kathleen

LEGAL NOTICES

COPYRIGHT

DISCLAIMER

TABLE OF CONTENTS

INTRODUCTION

Living healthy and staying fit is a necessary prerequisites to long life in this world. And we cannot be healthy if we continue to consume foods that will impact negatively on our health. Most of the foods being sold out there are laden with food additives and chemicals which experts has warned has not be confirmed to be safe for our body. Hence a need to watch what we consume and go on a program that will restore our body food relationship in a healthy way.

Whole Food Diet emphasizes eating of whole natural foods. This book "30 Day Whole Food Challenge: Over 100 Delicious Whole Food Recipes to Lose Weight and Stay Fit" is written to guide you by explaining the basics of this type of diet, the benefits and how you can prepare these dishes that are not only delicious but also healthy.

You cannot compromise your health and life at the expense of just anyhow food, be it fast foods, junks etc. Learn how to live healthy by going on Whole Food Diet. It will definitely change your life.

Amanda Kathleen

CHAPTER ONE

AN OVERVIEW

What Is Whole Food Diet?

It means a diet plan that emphasizes the consumption of foods that are still in their raw natural state. These are foods that still looks as they did growing in nature, or very close to it. Basically, foods that has not been tampered with, and no chemicals or preservatives have been added.

The human body runs most efficiently on food that is in its natural form, or very close to it. When we made the body to work on processed foods, we are making the body's job harder in processing those foods and if the body's job is made easier, life will be easy for us as we will live healthy.

What are Whole foods?

Whole food refers to produce of any kind like:
- Whole grains (rice, whole wheat, oats, millet, quinoa, barley etc)
- Fresh vegetables such as cucumbers, leafy greens, avocados, squash, radishes, carrots, and sweet potatoes
- Fresh or dried fruit such as oranges, grapes, apples, pears, watermelon, tomatoes, mangoes, pineapple, strawberries, and bananas
- Dairy products that does not contain any added sugar or chemical flavorings such as plain greek yogurt
- Meat, fish and poultry that is baked, roasted, grilled, or boiled
- Nuts and legumes and products made from them, for example hummus and nut butter as long as there is no chemicals, added sugar, or unhealthy fats.

The following does not constitute Whole food
- Foods with too many ingredients, chemical additives, or ingredients that you can't pronounce
- Processed food products such as: crackers, rehydrated mashed potatoes, or cookies snack bars and candy, prepared soups and frozen dinners/desserts, most boxed cereals and breads, jarred spaghetti and pizza sauces, and yogurts
- Most refrigerated prepared foods and condiments.

How It Works?

As much as possible you must avoid foods laden with chemicals and preservatives and get your nutritional requirements from natural food sources. However please note that plants based food begins to deteriorate as soon as they are detach from their life-source, so it is advisable to eat whole fruits and vegetables within a day or thereabout of picking them or buying them to get the most nutritional benefits from them. Frozen whole fruits and vegetables can also be a nutritious choice, as they are flash-frozen very soon after picking.

Here is a sample meal guide for your whole food diet plan. It is advisable to consume a variety of whole foods throughout the day to adequately meet your body's nutrient needs.

Breakfast
- You may eat whole-grain bread with real cheese, stay away from boxed cereals, instant oatmeal and commercial pastries.
- You can also eat cottage cheese and fruit, plain yogurt with natural milk, and eggs.
- A bowl of cut-up fruit and/or cooked whole-grains (brown rice, quinoa, etc.) with almond or soy milk.

Lunch
- You can grill, bake or roast your choice of food for the day be it pork, chicken, beef or seafood, vegetables can also be included in your main course.
- Burrito bowl with avocado

- Green salad with a variety of veggies and beans,
- Curry or stir-fried entree with brown rice
- A bowl of hearty vegetable soup.
- Sandwiches on whole-grain bread

Dinner

- Baked potatoes or winter squash topped with raw and/or cooked vegetables, or a hearty chili.
- Whole grain pasta with fresh tomato sauce and vegetables
- Roasted squash, eggplant or Portabello mushroom over salad
- Homemade soup or chili

Snacks

Snacks are allow in Whole food diet. Below are various snacks that can be consumed
- Dairy: cheese, yogurt, hard-boiled eggs
- Fruits such as apples, pears, melon, grapefruit, orange, dried fruit
- Vegetables such as kale chips, carrots, avocado, celery, bell pepper, zucchini
- Nuts such as pistachios, almonds, cashews, trail mix, nut butters
- Snack bars made from whole food ingredients (e.g. KIND)
- Beans such as black beans, edamame, lentils, and hummus
- Avoid potato chips, energy bars and sugary beverages like soda.

Whole foods can be gotten from local farmers markets and farm stands. Grocery stores also sell whole foods, although they will not be as fresh as what you'll find at farmers markets. A search online for "farmers markets," "produce stands," and "CSAs" (community supported agriculture) near you will help you to locate the freshest local produce.

Benefits of Whole Food Diet

- The focus of this diet is whole food. It requires no extra money that will be spent on special diet foods. All you need for this program is readily available at your local grocery store or at the farmers market.

- By taking enough sleep, water, vegetables and fruits your skin will be looking brighter and younger and your hair will be also shining.
- By eliminating packaged and processed foods from your diets help you to stay away from ailments caused by food additives and chemicals and also keep you fit. Junk foods and fast foods has not in any way been beneficial to our body's health.
- Whole foods, vegetables and fruits are rich in nutrients like calcium, fiber, magnesium, B vitamins, protein, Vitamin D, essential fatty acids and potassium that the body needs to keep itself in top shape.
- They are full of good fats, this eliminates the consumption of trans fats and saturated fats from your diet that are not beneficial to your health.
- Most whole foods like whole grains, fruits, vegetables, nuts, seeds, legumes, and beans are full of fiber which aids digestion and regularity. Fiber reduces the risk of diabetes, helps to lower cholesterol, protect against heart diseases and keep the intestinal tracts healthy and functioning properly.
- Whole foods supply more energy to the body. They energize and keep the bodies from having to break down foods like animal products that are related to cancer, diabetes and poor heart health.

Challenges

- It requires a lot of effort to carry out and highly restrictive. A lot of adjustment in terms of meal preparation, grocery shopping (always checking the labels for restricted contents) will be required.
- Self-prepared food could be time-demanding and requires a lot of energy. But self-prepared foods are free from chemicals and additives which prevent you from lots of health problems.
- It is sometimes very expensive to consume whole foods. This is one of the side effect, but you also have to know that eating of processed foods can at the same time cause ailment and disease to your body.
- Making transition from your old diet to this diet might cause digestive issues. This should not cause worry as the body need time to adjust to this new diet.

If you experience digestive issue, the following tips will help you to overcome the problem,

- Take smaller bites and make sure you chew your food thoroughly

- Eat plenty of fruits and vegetables

- Don't get too full

- Eat balanced meals

- Increase vegetable and fiber intake gradually

- Eat foods with probiotics

- Soak your beans before eating

- Eliminate wheat and dairy from your food

- Avoid fake sugars

- Reduce intake of fresh and dried fruit intake

The following tips will help you to succeed while undergoing this diet program.
- Make use of whole wheat flour instead of white flour
- Always check your labels before you buy any food products for ingredients, chemical additives, or ingredients that you can't pronounce
- It is advisable to always cook your food to avoid accidental eating at eateries. Eating at eateries will not help you as you won't know if those ingredients are whole food compliant.
- Avoid foods not on your diets from friends during your whole food diet program.
- Think natural whole foods. Cook using fruit, peppers, onions, fresh herbs, and other foods with inherently strong flavor notes to season your food.
- Learn to make leftovers. Preparing these recipes could be laboring and stressful atimes. It is advisable to make extra so you have leftovers.
- Buy food that are in season. This will help you to save money.
- Make use of slow cooker to save more time. This helps because all you need is just to dump the food items into it while you wait for it to cook on its own. This saves time in cooking.

30 Day Whole Food Challenge

This means for 30 days your focus is on whole food and cut back on processed foods. Over these 30 days, it will help you to save money, eat healthier, feel better and lose weight.

Like we've discussed above this challenge means embracing whole foods like vegetables, fruits and whole grains, plus healthy proteins and fats. It also means cutting back on refined grains, added sugar, additives, preservatives, unhealthy fats and large amounts of salt.

If you are ready to for this challenge please read on as I explain in detail, step by step on how to prepare these delicious meal both for breakfast, lunch, snacks and diner.

CHAPTER TWO

BREAKFAST RECIPES

APPLE CINNAMON TOAST

Yields: 4 servings
Serving Size: 1 bowl
Preparation Time: 10 minutes
Cooking Time: 8 hours
Total Time: 8 hours and 10 minutes

INGREDIENTS

- ¾ cup half-and-half
- 1 ¾ tsp. ground cinnamon
- 8 slices whole grain bread, sliced into halves
- 5 eggs, beaten
- ¾ cup milk
- ¼ tsp. fine sea salt
- Cooking spray
- 3 apples, peeled, cored and sliced
- 4 tbsp. brown sugar, divided

COOKING INSTRUCTIONS

1. First spray cooking oil unto your slow cooker pot.
2. Sequence the layer of bread.
3. Top this layer with the apple slices.
4. Take the eggs (first pour half egg then half), milk, salt, cinnamon and three tablespoons of the brown sugar and mingle well.
5. Pour this mixture on the top of the apple slices.

6. Sprinkle the remaining brown sugar on top.
7. Seal the pot properly.
8. Cook on low temperature for 6 to 8 hours.
9. Let it cool before serving.

BREAKFAST QUINOA

Yields: 5 servings
Serving Size: 1 cup
Preparation Time: 5 minutes
Cooking Time: 2 hours
Total Time: 2 hours and 5 minutes

INGREDIENTS

- 4 dates, chopped
- 1 apple, peeled, cored and diced
- 1 tsp. vanilla extract
- 2 tsp. cinnamon
- ¼ tsp. salt
- 3 cups almond milk
- ¼ tsp. nutmeg
- 1 cup quinoa
- ¼ cup pepitas

COOKING INSTRUCTIONS

1. Place all the ingredients in a slow cooker.
2. Set it on high temperature.
3. Then cook it for 2 hours.
4. Serve it while warm.

ORANGE CINNAMON ROLLS

Yields: 12 servings
Serving Size: 1 roll
Preparation Time: 15 minutes
Cooking Time: 30 minutes
Total Time: 45 minutes

INGREDIENTS

- 4 tbsp. butter, divided
- 1 egg, beaten
- ¼ oz. package active dry yeast
- 1 ½ cup whole wheat pastry flour
- 4 tsp. ground cinnamon
- 2 tbsp. orange juice, divided
- ½ tsp. sea salt
- ½ tsp. orange zest, grated
- 1 cup powdered sugar, sifted
- 1 ½ cup all-purpose flour
- ¾ cup nonfat milk, warmed
- ¾ cup brown sugar, divided

COOKING INSTRUCTIONS

1. Blend and mingle correctly yeast, milk and 2 tablespoon brown sugar in a bowl.
2. Leave it for about 10 minutes.
3. Add 2 tablespoons butter and egg into the yeast concoction. And mix very well.
4. In another bowl mix both flour, orange zest, juice and salt.
5. Fold this into the main mixture.
6. Knead (work with hands) for about 5 minutes.
7. Coat muffin pan with a little bit of butter.
8. Make a rectangle from the dough.
9. In a small bowl, combine the cinnamon and the remaining brown sugar.
10. Then place it in the refrigerator overnight.
11. Bake in the oven at 350* F for 18-20 minutes.

12. Decorate (dust) with powdered sugar before serving.

BREAKFAST BURRITO

Prep Time: 5 minutes
Cook Time: 5 minutes
Total Time: 10 minutes
Serving Size: 1

INGREDIENTS

- ¼ cup chopped veggies (spinach, black olives, bell pepper, tomato, etc)
- Sliced Ham (It should be large enough to fold and of medium-thickness so that it doesn't break when wrapped. More than one slice will be required)
- 2 eggs (or egg whites)
- Salsa, Guacamole, Cilantro can be used but they are optional.

COOKING INSTRUCTIONS

1. Saute the veggies in a small bit of oil over medium high heat.
2. Then whisk the eggs in a small bowl and pour over the mixed veggie.
3. With the aid of a spatula, scramble the mixture until well cooked. Once done transfer the eggs out of the pan.
4. Then roll the ham around the eggs and return onto the skillet.
5. Grill for a few seconds each side until the ham is slightly brown.
6. You can now serve with salsa, guacamole, and a sprig of fresh cilantro on top.

PANCAKE & SAUSAGE

Yields: 16 servings
Serving Size: 1 slice
Preparation Time: 15 minutes
Cooking Time: 40 minutes
Total Time: 55 minutes

INGREDIENTS

- 2 cups nonfat milk
- ¾ cup pecans, chopped
- 3 cups pancake mix
- 2 apples, peeled, cored and sliced
- ¼ cup maple syrup
- 1 lb. pre-cooked breakfast sausage links chopped Cooking spray
- 3 eggs
- 1 tsp. ground ginger

COOKING INSTRUCTIONS

1. Preheat your oven up to 350*F.
2. Coat baking skillet with cooking oil spinkles.
3. In a bowl, blend the eggs, ginger and milk.
4. Get another bowl, combine the pecans and pancake and mix well.
5. Add the first mixture into the second mixture and add half of the apples and sausages.
6. Pour mixture into a baking pan.
7. Adorn the remaining apples and sausages into it and bake for about 40 minutes.
8. Top with the maple syrup before serving.

CHOCOLATE CHIA & FRESH BERRY PUDDING

Yields: 4 servings
Serving Size: 1 cup
Preparation Time: 5 minutes
Cooking Time: 30 minutes
Total Time: 35 minutes

INGREDIENTS

- ½ cup fresh blueberries, chopped
- 2 cups milk
- ½ cup chia seeds
- 2 tbsp. maple syrup
- ½ cup fresh raspberries, chopped
- 2 tbsp. cocoa powder
- ½ cup fresh blackberries, chopped

COOKING INSTRUCTIONS

1. First put all the ingredients in a bowl and mix it well.
2. Then Chill in the refrigerator for 1 to 2 hours.
3. When it becomes properly cool then serve it.

AVOCADO BAKED EGG

Prep Time: 5mins
Cook Time: 15mins
Total Time: 20mins

- 1/2 lemon, squeezed
- 1 avocado
- Sea salt and pepper
- 2 eggs

COOKING INSTRUCTIONS

1. Preheat your oven to 425°F.
2. Scoop out the inside of the Avocado leaving half inch rim.
3. Break the egg into the avocado and place on a baking sheet. Then Sprinkle lemon juice, salt, and pepper over both Avocado halves.
4. Then Bake for 15 minutes or until the yolks set.
5. You can put some foil on your cookie sheet for a much easier clean up!

TORTILLA BREAKFAST STRATA

Yields: 12 servings
Serving Size: 1 bowl
Preparation Time: 20 minutes
Cooking Time: 50 minutes
Total Time: 1 hour and 10 minutes

INGREDIENTS

- 4 oz. canned green chili, diced
- 1 tbsp. olive oil
- 8 eggs
- 6 whole wheat tortillas
- 2 cups Monterey Jack cheese, grated
- ¾ lb. leafy greens, roughly chopped

- 2 cups low fat milk
- 14 oz. package sausage, chopped
- ¾ tsp. fine sea salt

COOKING INSTRUCTIONS

1. First put olive oil in a skillet on medium heat.
2. Brown the sausage into olive oil for about 10 minutes.
3. Then remove it from the pan and drain.
4. Put the leafy greens in the pan and toss until soft and wilted for about 6 minutes.
5. In a bowl, mix the milk, eggs and salt properly.
6. Coat the casserole dish with a little bit of oil.
7. Place half of the tortillas inside it.
8. Pour on the top with half of the cheese, half of the leafy greens and half of chili.
9. Pour half of the eggs mixture into it.
10. Repeat layer using the same procedure.
11. Chill (make cool) in the refrigerator for 2 hours.
12. Bake in the oven at 350* F for 50 minutes.

CARAMEL OATMEAL

Yields: 6 servings
Serving Size: 1 bowl
Preparation Time: 5 minutes
Cooking Time: 2 hours
Total Time: 2 hours and 5 minutes

INGREDIENTS

- ¼ tsp. nutmeg
- 4 apples, sliced thinly
- 7 cups almond milk
- 1 ½ tsp. cinnamon

- ¼ tsp. ginger
- 10 dates, soaked in water for half an hour
- ¼ cup maple syrup
- 2 cups steel cut oats

COOKING INSTRUCTIONS

1. First put the apples, cinnamon, oats, almond milk, nutmeg and ginger in a slow cooker.
2. Set it on high and cook for 3 hours.
3. While waiting, put the dates and maple syrup in a blender and blend it properly.
4. Blend it until the consistency has become smooth.
5. Serve the maple and date mixture with the cooked oats.

BAKED APPLE & CINNAMON

Yields: 6 servings
Serving Size: 1 slice
Preparation Time: 10 minutes
Cooking Time: 25 minutes
Total Time: 35 minutes

INGREDIENTS

- 1 ½ tsp. cinnamon
- ½ tsp. sea salt
- 2 cups quinoa, cooked
- 2 eggs, beaten
- ¼ tsp. nutmeg
- ¼ tsp. ginger
- 10 dates, pitted and soaked in water for half an hour
- 1 apple, grated
- ½ cup unsweetened applesauce
- 1 tsp. baking soda

COOKING INSTRUCTIONS

1. First preheat your oven up to 350*F.
2. Then put the dates into a strainer to drain the water from it.
3. Put the quinoa and dates in a food processor and beat the pulses until well blend.
4. Add the rest of the ingredients into it.
5. Put some more pulses on it.
6. Then pour all this mixture into a baking pan.
7. Bake the mixture for 25 minutes.
8. Allow it to cool and make slices of it before serving.

ALMOND & BLUEBERRY SCONE

Yields: 8 servings
Serving Size: 1 slice
Preparation Time: 10 minutes
Cooking Time: 30 minutes
Total Time: 40 minutes

INGREDIENTS

- 1 ¼ cups raw cashews
- 1 tsp. vanilla extract
- 1 cup fresh blueberries
- 1 tsp. baking powder
- ¼ cup maple syrup
- 1 tsp. almond extract
- ¼ cup coconut oil
- 2 eggs, beaten
- ½ tsp. sea salt
- ¼ cup arrowroot powder

COOKING INSTRUCTIONS

1. First preheat your oven to 350*F.
2. Crush the cashews in a food processor until it become powder.
3. Pour the cashew powder into a bowl.
4. Add the rest of the dry ingredients into it.
5. In another bowl combine the wet ingredients.
6. Then mingle this mixture into the first bowl.
7. Pour the mixture into a baking pan and bake for 30 minutes.
8. Let it cool before slicing and serving.

SWEET POTATO WAFFLES

Yields: 6 servings
Serving Size: 1 to 2 waffles
Preparation Time: 10 minutes
Cooking Time: 10 minutes
Total Time: 20 minutes

INGREDIENTS

- ½ cup ham, diced
- 2 tsp. baking powder
- 1 cup sweet potato purée
- 1 ½ cup whole wheat pastry flour
- ½ tsp. sea salt
- ¼ cup cornstarch
- 1 cup buttermilk
- Cooking spray
- 2 tbsp. brown sugar
- ¼ tsp. nutmeg, grated
- 2 eggs
- 4 tbsp. butter, melted

COOKING INSTRUCTIONS

1. First preheat your waffle iron.
2. Then mingle the cornstarch, baking powder, flour, brown sugar, nutmeg and salt in a bowl.
3. In a distinct bowl take eggs, butter, sweet potato purée and buttermilk and whisk it appropriately.
4. Pour this collection of eggs, butter, sweet potato puree and butter milk into the first mixture.
5. Add the ham slices into it and shower your waffle iron with cooking oil.
6. Then pour enough batter (mixture of all ingredients) in it.

SPINACH OMELET

Yields: 8 servings
Serving Size: 1 omelet
Preparation Time: 5 minutes
Cooking Time: 15 minutes
Total Time: 20 minutes

INGREDIENTS

- 2 tsp. baking powder
- ½ cup nutritional yeast
- ½ tsp. sea salt
- 4 cups spinach, chopped
- 2 cups chickpea flour
- ⅓ cup water
- 3 tbsp. flax meal
- 2 tsp. turmeric
- 1 tsp. garlic powder

COOKING INSTRUCTIONS

1. First put all the dry ingredients except spinach in a bowl.
2. Mix to blend well.
3. Put ⅓ of the mixture in a pan and cook it on mid heat.
4. Add water into it.
5. Then mix it very well.
6. Add a little of the spinach into the batter (mixture).
7. Cook it for 5 to 7 minutes from each side.
8. Serve it with the remaining spinach.

SOUTHWESTERN AVOCADO TOAST

Yields: 4 servings
Serving Size: 1 piece
Preparation Time: 10 minutes
Cooking Time: 3 minutes
Total Time: 13 minutes

INGREDIENTS

- 3 tomatoes, diced
- 1 tbsp. cilantro, chopped
- ½ cup onion, diced
- 2 tbsp. freshly squeezed lime juice
- 2 avocados, mashed
- Pinch of sea salt
- 1 clove garlic, minced

COOKING INSTRUCTIONS

1. First combine all the ingredients in a bowl except bread and avocado. And mix it well.

2. Toast the bread until it becomes golden brown.
3. Spread a layer of the mashed avocados and the mixture of other ingredients on each slice.
4. Place the slices in a plate properly and then serve it.

CINNAMON TOAST CRUNCH

Yields: 1 serving
Serving Size: 1 cup
Preparation Time: 1 hour and 15 minutes
Cooking Time: 30 minutes
Total Time: 1 hour and 45 minutes

INGREDIENTS

- ¼ cup applesauce
- 1 tsp. vanilla extract
- 2 eggs, beaten
- ¼ cup almond milk
- ¼ cup brown sugar
- ¼ tsp. baking powder
- 1 cup sorghum flour
- 1 cup oat flour
- 1 tsp. cinnamon
- ¼ cup coconut oil

COOKING INSTRUCTIONS

1. First preheat your oven up to 350* F.
2. Put the 2 flours, brown sugar, baking powder and cinnamon in a mixing bowl and mix well.
3. Then get another bowl and mix the rest of the ingredients.

4. After then mix the two mixtures together and mix them properly.
5. Wrap dough in cling wrap and chill in the refrigerator for 1 hour.
6. Roll the dough as thinly as possible and press firmly into a baking pan.
7. Bake it in the oven for 30 minutes, flipping halfway through it.
8. Use a pizza cutter to make slices of it and then serve it.

PUMPKIN COCONUT SMOOTHIE

Prep Time: 5mins
Total Time: 5mins
Servings: 2 servings

INGREDIENTS

- 1 cup coconut milk
- 2 teaspoons pumpkin pie spice (can be substituted for cinnamon and ginger)
- 1 cup ice
- 1 frozen banana sliced
- 1/4 cup organic pumpkin puree
- One scoop of collagen powder can be added for more protein

COOKING INSTRUCTIONS

1. First of all add coconut milk, pumpkin pie spice, pumpkin, banana, and ice to Blendtec or Vitamix.
2. Blend on smoothie cycle or high speed until it is smooth.

BAKED FRENCH TOAST

Yields: 8 servings
Serving Size: 1 piece
Preparation Time: 15 minutes
Cooking Time: 25 minutes
Total Time: 40 minutes

INGREDIENTS

- ½ tsp. orange zest, grated
- ¼ cup freshly squeezed orange juice
- 8 slices whole grain bread, sliced into sticks
- ¾ cup milk
- ¾ cup maple syrup
- 4 eggs
- ¼ tsp. nutmeg, grated
- 1 tsp. vanilla extract
- ¼ tsp. sea salt
- Cooking spray

COOKING INSTRUCTIONS

1. First preheat your oven up to 375*F
2. Spray baking pan with cooking oil.
3. Put the orange zest, orange juice and maple syrup into a stove-top pan.
4. Bring to a boil and then (stay) for 10 minutes.
5. In a bowl merge the milk, eggs, nutmeg, vanilla extract and sea salt correctly.
6. Then dunk each slice of bread into the concoction.
7. Arrange these slices on the baking pan and bake for 15 minutes.
8. Drizzle with the maple-orange syrup before serving.

APPLES & PEARS WITH QUINOA

Yields: 1 serving
Serving Size: 1 cup
Preparation Time: 30 minutes
Cooking Time: 4 hours
Total Time: 4 hours and 30 minutes

INGREDIENTS

- 2 tsp. cinnamon
- ¼ tsp. ginger
- 5 pears, cored and sliced
- ½ cup water
- 1 cup quinoa, cooked
- 1 tsp. vanilla extract
- 5 apples, cored and sliced
- ¼ tsp. nutmeg
- ¼ tsp. cloves

COOKING INSTRUCTIONS

1. First put all the ingredients except the quinoa in slow cooker.
2. Switch it to high temperature.
3. Then Cook it for about 4 hours.
4. Allow the mixture cool after then.
5. Put the mixture and the quinoa and pulses in the blender and blend it until its consistency becomes smooth.
6. Chill it in the refrigerator before serving.

CHAPTER THREE

SEAFOOD RECIPES

SEAFOOD WITH POTATOES AND KALE

Yields: 4 servings
Serving Size: 1 bowl
Preparation Time: 10 minutes
Cooking Time: 25 minutes
Total Time: 35 minutes

INGREDIENTS

- 1 ½ lb. halibut fillets, cut into big chunks
- 12 sea scallops
- 1 cup kale, chopped
- 4 potatoes, quarter cut
- 6 cups reduced sodium chicken stock
- ¼ tsp. fine sea salt
- 2 tbsp. olive oil, divided
- 1 leek, white portion sliced thinly
- ¼ tsp. freshly ground black pepper

COOKING INSTRUCTIONS

1. Pour half of the olive oil into a pot on mid heat.
2. Then add the green onion and cook it for 8 minutes.
3. Add the kale, potatoes and make thin soup.
4. Simmer for 10 minutes.
5. Add fish in it and simmer for 12 minutes.

6. Sprinkle the scallops with salt and pepper.
7. Put down the remaining oil into the skillet.
8. Cook the scallops in the pot for about 2 to 3 minutes on each side.
9. Ladle it into bowls and serve while warm.

BAKED SALMON WITH MANGO SALSA

Yields: 4 servings
Serving Size: 1 salmon fillet and 1 tbsp. salsa
Preparation Time: 5 minutes
Cooking Time: 6 minutes
Total Time: 11 minutes

INGREDIENTS

- 1 ½ tbsp. lime juice
- 1 ½ tsp. vegetable oil
- 1 shallot, chopped
- ¼ tsp. black pepper
- 1 tsp. fine sea salt, divided
- 1 jalapeño pepper, seeded and chopped
- ½ cup cilantro
- 4 salmon fillets
- 2 mangoes, peeled and diced

COOKING INSTRUCTIONS

1. Preheat your oven up to 425* F.
2. Then, in a bowl mix together the vegetable oil with the pepper and half of the salt.
3. Coat all sides of the fish with the vegetable oil blend.
4. Put down the fish fillet in a baking pan.
5. Bake for 5-6 minutes.

6. In a mixing bowl, blend the jalapeño, mangoes, lime juice, shallot and remaining salt.
7. Serve the salmon with the mango-salsa mixture and cilantro.

BAKED CRISPY COD

Yields: 4 servings
Serving Size: 1 cod fillet
Preparation Time: 10 minutes
Cooking Time: 12 minutes
Total Time: 22 minutes

INGREDIENTS

- 4 cod fillets (skinless)
- 2 tbsp. lemon juice, divided
- ¼ cup whole wheat breadcrumbs
- 3 tbsp. parsley, chopped
- ¾ tsp. fine sea salt
- 2 tbsp. chives, chopped
- ¼ tsp. freshly ground black pepper
- Cooking spray
- 3 tbsp. butter, melted and divided

COOKING INSTRUCTIONS

1. First preheat your oven up to 425*F.
2. Coat the baking pan with cooking oil.
3. Season the cod with the salt and pepper.
4. Sprinkle half of the melted butter over the cod.
5. Trickle with half of the lemon sap.
6. In a mixing bowl, blend the parsley, breadcrumbs, and chives.

7. Season the cod with this mixture.
8. Sprinkle with the remaining lemon sap and butter and bake in the oven for about 10 - 12 minutes.

BAKED TUNA WITH SPINACH & STRAWBERRY SALSA

Yields: 4 servings
Serving Size: 1 small plate
Preparation Time: 10 minutes
Cooking Time: 22 minutes
Total Time: 32 minutes

INGREDIENTS

- 2 tbsp. freshly squeezed lemon juice, divided
- 4 tuna fillets (boneless and skinless)
- 1 lb. strawberries, diced
- 2 kiwis, diced
- 2 tbsp. fresh mint leaves, chopped
- 1 lb. baby spinach leaves
- 1 jalapeño pepper, minced
- 1 tsp. lemon zest
- 1 cucumber, diced

COOKING INSTRUCTIONS

1. First preheat your oven up to 350*F.
2. Then carefully arrange the tuna fillets on a baking pan.
3. Splash the lemon rind over the fillets.
4. Bake for 15 minutes.
5. In a bowl, mix together the cucumber, strawberries, jalapeño, kiwis, mint, and half of the lemon sap.

6. Take oil in a skillet on mid heat.
7. And add the spinach and cook for 5 to 7 minutes.
8. Then add the remaining lemon juice to it.
9. Put the spinach into four plates.
10. Add on top of it, the tuna fillets and salsa before serving.

CLAMS WITH SUN-DRIED TOMATOES

Yields: 4 servings
Serving Size: 1 bowl
Preparation Time: 10 minutes
Cooking Time: 26 minutes
Total Time: 36 minutes

INGREDIENTS

- ½ cup sun-dried tomatoes, sliced
- 24 clams, scrubbed, rinsed and drained
- 2 tbsp. parsley, chopped
- 1 onion, sliced thinly
- 5 cloves garlic, sliced thinly
- ⅛ tsp. fine sea salt
- 2 tsp. extra virgin olive oil
- ⅛ tsp. red chili flakes, crushed
- ½ cup dry white wine

COOKING INSTRUCTIONS

1. Pour the oil into a large skillet on mid heat.
2. Fry the onion until slightly brown for about 10 minutes.
3. Add unto it, the garlic, salt and chili flakes and Cook for 1 minute.
4. Add the tomatoes and wine into it.
5. Bring it to a boil and simmer it for 3 to 5 minutes.

6. Add in the clams. Cover and let it cook for 10 minutes.
7. Then remove the clams that did not open up.
8. Ladle (spoon) it into soup bowls.
9. Garnish it with parsley before serving.

CATFISH IN COCONUT CURRY

Yields: 4 servings
Serving Size: 1 cup
Preparation Time: 10 minutes
Cooking Time: 21 minutes
Total Time: 31 minutes

INGREDIENTS

- 1 ¼ lb. white fish fillet, cut into cubes
- 5 cups baby spinach leaves
- ¼ cup fresh cilantro leaves
- 2 tbsp. lime juice
- 1 ½ tbsp. red curry paste
- 1 tsp. sugar
- 1 tbsp. coconut oil
- 1 white onion, sliced thinly
- 1 cup coconut milk
- ¼ tsp. fine sea salt
- 1 tbsp. fish sauce

COOKING INSTRUCTIONS

1. First add the oil to a deep skillet on medium heat.
2. Then put the onion in oil and cook for 6 minutes.
3. Mix the red curry paste, sugar, coconut milk and salt.
4. Mix it thoroughly and simmer.

5. Add the fish, fish sauce and spinach.
6. And cook for 15 minutes.

Garnish with the cilantro and shower with the lime sap before serving.

GRILLED FISH WITH OLIVE & PARSLEY

Yields: 4 servings
Serving Size: 1 fish fillet and 1 tablespoon salsa
Preparation Time: 10 minutes
Cooking Time: 10 minutes
Total Time: 20 minutes

INGREDIENTS

- 1 tbsp. fresh oregano
- 1 tbsp. extra virgin olive oil
- ¾ lb. monkfish fillets, butterfly-cut
- 1 tbsp. freshly squeezed lemon juice
- ½ cup parsley
- ¼ tsp. fine sea salt
- ¼ tsp. ground black pepper
- 1 cup olives, pitted

COOKING INSTRUCTIONS

1. Rub the salt and pepper onto the fish fillets.
2. Chill in the refrigerator for 2 hours.
3. First preheat your grill.
4. Then put the lemon juice, parsley, olives and oregano in a food processor.
5. And pulse until well blended but still a little chunky.
6. Use paper towels to dry the fish.
7. Brush it with the oil.

8. Grill the fish for 8 to 10 minutes.

9. Serve it with salsa.

SPAGHETTI WITH SARDINES & PINE NUTS

Yields: 4 servings
Serving Size: 1 bowl
Preparation Time: 15 minutes
Cooking Time: 15 minutes
Total Time: 30 minutes

INGREDIENTS

- ½ onion, diced
- ¾ cup parsley, chopped
- 8 oz. whole wheat spaghetti, cooked according to package directions
- 2 tbsp. red wine vinegar
- ¼ cup pine nuts, toasted
- ¼ tsp. fine sea salt
- ¼ tsp. freshly ground black pepper
- 2 tbsp. orange juice
- 3 tbsp. dried currants
- 4 oz. sardines in olive oil
- 1 tbsp. extra virgin olive oil

COOKING INSTRUCTIONS

1. In a bowl, mix the orange juice and currants and set aside.
2. Get the oil from the sardines and pour into the skillet.
3. Add the extra virgin olive oil.
4. Sauté the onion for 5 minutes.
5. Then add the sardines and mash with the onion.
6. Sprinkle the salt and pepper to season.

7. Toss the spaghetti over it.
8. Add the currants and orange juice, along with the vinegar and pine nuts.
9. Garnish it with the pine nuts before serving.

SPINACH & TURBOT GRATIN

Yields: 4 servings
Serving Size: 1 slice
Preparation Time: 30 minutes
Cooking Time: 30 minutes
Total Time: 60 minutes

INGREDIENTS

- 1 cup half-and-half
- ½ tsp. nutmeg, grated
- 2 cloves garlic, chopped
- ¼ cup fresh chives, chopped and divided
- ½ tsp. fine sea salt
- 16 oz. spinach
- 1 ½ tbsp. butter, divided
- ¾ lb. turbot fillets (boneless and skinless)
- 1 ½ tbsp. whole wheat bread crumbs
- 1 shallot, chopped
- 1 tbsp. all-purpose flour
- ¼ tsp. ground white pepper

COOKING INSTRUCTIONS

1. First preheat your oven to 400* F.
2. Grease the baking dish with a little bit of the butter.

3. Melt the remaining butter in a skillet on medium heat.

4. And cook the fish for 5 minutes.

5. Transfer the fish into a serving platter and cover it with foil to keep warm.

6. In the same skillet, add the garlic and shallot and cook for 4 minutes.

7. Then add the flour and cook for another minute.

8. Add the salt, pepper, half-and-half and nutmeg. Simmer it for 2 minutes.

9. Get a large mixing bowl, mix the spinach, cooked fish and chives together

10. Add this to the garlic and shallot mixture. Blend it well.

11. Spread all the mixture onto a baking dish.

12. Give upper coat with the breadcrumbs.

13. Bake it for 15 minutes.

14. Let it cool a little and slice it before serving.

SCALLOPS WITH TARRAGON SAUCE

Yields: 6 servings
Serving Size: 1 bowl
Preparation Time: 10 minutes
Cooking Time: 10 minutes
Total Time: 20 minutes

INGREDIENTS

- ½ tsp. ground black pepper
- 1 tbsp. extra-virgin olive oil
- 1 ½ lb. wild-caught sea scallops
- 2 tbsp. rice vinegar
- 2 shallots, chopped
- 2 cups fresh cherries, pitted and quarter cut
- 1 tbsp. tarragon, chopped
- ½ tsp. fine sea salt

COOKING INSTRUCTIONS

1. First dry the scallops using paper towels before seasoning with the salt and pepper.
2. In a pot, pour the oil into it and wait till it becomes very hot before adding the scallops.
3. Let it sear until lightly brown on both sides.
4. Transfer these to a serving platter. Cover with foil to keep warm.
5. Reduce the heat and put the shallots in the skillet.
6. Cook for about 2 minutes.
7. Add the cherries and vinegar into it.
8. Cook for more 5 minutes.
9. Pour the cherry mixture over the scallops and sprinkle it with the tarragon before serving.

SALMON TERIYAKI WITH RICE

Yields: 4 servings
Serving Size: 1 bowl
Preparation Time: 10 minutes
Cooking Time: 30 minutes
Total Time: 40 minutes

INGREDIENTS

- 14 oz. mixed frozen vegetables 4 tbsp. teriyaki sauce, divided
- 4 salmon fillets (boneless and skinless)
- 4 cups brown rice, cooked
- 1 tsp. olive oil

COOKING INSTRUCTIONS

1. First preheat your oven up to 350*F.
2. Then lay the salmon fillets on a baking pan.

3. Shower with 1 tablespoon teriyaki sauce.
4. And bake for 20 minutes.
5. While waiting, pour the oil into a skillet on medium heat.
6. Add the frozen vegetables into it.
7. Stir very well until the vegetables are a little soft but still firm.
8. Add brown rice in it and mix well.
9. Then add the remaining teriyaki sauce.
10. Put the rice in four bowls.
11. Garnish with the salmon and serve.

CHAPTER FOUR

SALAD RECIPES

CELERY & ALMOND SALAD

Yields: 6 servings
Serving Size: 1 bowl
Preparation Time: 15 minutes
Cooking Time: 0 minutes
Total Time: 15 minutes

INGREDIENTS

- 2 tbsp. lemon zest
- ¾ tsp. red chili flakes, crushed
- 2 oz. dates, pitted
- ½ cup parsley, chopped
- ¼ cup fresh mint, chopped
- ½ cup hot water
- ½ cup celery, sliced thinly
- ¼ cup whole almonds, toasted and chopped
- 2 tbsp. tahini
- ¼ cup freshly squeezed lemon juice
- ¼ tsp. fine sea salt

COOKING INSTRUCTIONS

1. Take the dates in a bowl.
2. And soak in hot water for 10 minutes.
3. Then transfer the dates and liquid to your blender.

4. Add the tahini, lemon juice, lemon zest, salt and chili flakes.
5. Blend until smooth.
6. Toss with the parsley, mint and celery.
7. Garnish with the almonds before serving.

MEDITERRANEAN SALAD

Yields: 4 servings
Serving Size: 1 bowl
Preparation Time: 30 minutes to 1 hour
Cooking Time: 0 minutes
Total Time: 15 minutes

INGREDIENTS

- 3 tbsp. red wine vinegar
- 1 clove garlic, minced
- 15 oz. unsalted canned garbanzo beans, drained
- 1 tsp. fresh thyme, chopped
- 1 cup grape tomatoes, cut into halves
- 1 cup kale, stems removed and sliced
- ½ cup onion, chopped
- 1 cup broccoli florets
- 1 tbsp. fresh parsley, chopped
- 2 tbsp. Kalamata olives, chopped
- 1 cucumber, chopped

COOKING INSTRUCTIONS

1. Put all the ingredients in a large bowl.
2. Chill in the refrigerator for 30 minutes to 1 hour before serving.

KALE, AVOCADO & CARROT SALAD

Yields: 4 servings
Serving Size: 1 bowl
Preparation Time: 5 minutes
Cooking Time: 0 minutes
Total Time: 5 minutes

INGREDIENTS

- 2 tbsp. sesame seeds, toasted
- ¼ cup onion, sliced thinly
- ½ avocado, peeled, pitted and cut into cubes
- 2 tbsp. freshly squeezed lemon juice
- ½ tsp. low sodium soy sauce
- 2 cups carrots, grated
- 4 cups kale, stems removed and chopped finely

COOKING INSTRUCTIONS

1. Take all the ingredients in a large salad bowl.
2. Mash the avocado and mix it with the rest of the ingredients in the bowl.
3. Serve when chilled for sometime.

GREEN SALAD WITH LEMON MISO DRESSING

Yields: 8 servings
Serving Size: 1 cup
Preparation Time: 5 minutes
Cooking Time: 0 minutes
Total Time: 5 minutes

INGREDIENTS

- 3 tbsp. white miso paste
- 8 radishes, trimmed and sliced
- 8 cups lettuce leaves, chopped
- 1 ½ cup barley, cooked
- 3 tbsp. freshly squeezed lemon juice
- 15 oz. unsalted canned garbanzo beans, rinsed and drained
- 1 cucumber, sliced thinly
- 1 shallot, chopped finely
- 3 tbsp. unsweetened apple juice

COOKING INSTRUCTIONS

1. First take the lettuce, barley, garbanzo beans, cucumber and radishes in a large salad bowl.
2. In a smaller bowl, combine the shallots, apple juice, lemon juice and miso paste and mix well.
3. Drizzle the salad with the dressing before serving.

RADISH SALAD

Yields: 6 servings
Serving Size: 1 bowl
Preparation Time: 5 minutes
Cooking Time: 0 minutes
Total Time: 5 minutes

INGREDIENTS

- ¾ cup fresh mint leaves, sliced
- ¼ tsp. fine sea salt
- 3 tbsp. freshly squeezed lemon juice
- 1 tbsp. vinegar
- 2 ½ lb. kohlrabi, peeled and sliced thinly with mandolin
- 1 tbsp. honey
- 6 radishes, peeled and sliced thinly with mandolin

COOKING INSTRUCTIONS

1. Mix the honey, vinegar and lemon juice in a bowl.
2. Then mix the rest of the ingredients into the dressing.
3. And season with the salt before serving.

COUSCOUS SALAD

Yields: 8 servings
Serving Size: 1 salad bowl
Preparation Time: 10 minutes
Cooking Time: 0 minutes
Total Time: 10 minutes

INGREDIENTS

- 2 zucchini, sliced
- 1 ¼ cup hot water
- 1 cup whole wheat couscous
- ¼ cup parsley
- ⅛ tsp. fine sea salt
- ¼ cup tahini
- 5 tbsp. white wine vinegar
- 1 cup grape tomatoes, cut in half
- 15 oz. canned chickpeas, rinsed and drained

COOKING INSTRUCTIONS

1. Pour the water in a bowl.
2. Soak the couscous in it for 5 minutes.
3. Fluff with a fork.
4. Then in another bowl, mix the salt, tahini and vinegar.
5. In a salad bowl, toss the zucchini, chickpeas, tomatoes and couscous with the tahini dressing.
6. Garnish with parsley before serving.

SALMON SALAD

Yields: 4 servings
Serving Size: 1 salad plate
Preparation Time: 15 minutes
Cooking Time: 10 minutes
Total Time: 25 minutes

INGREDIENTS

- 6 cups baby kale
- ¾ lb. salmon fillet (skinless, boneless)
- 2 tbsp. pickled jalapeño peppers, chopped
- 1 avocado, pitted, peeled and chopped, divided
- 2 tbsp. freshly squeezed lemon juice

COOKING INSTRUCTIONS

1. First preheat your oven up to 400*F.
2. Cover your baking sheet with parchment.
3. Place the salmon fillets on the baking pan.
4. And bake for 10 minutes.
5. Fragment the flesh using a fork.
6. Mash the avocado with lemon juice.
7. Toss the kale into this mixture.
8. And put the kale and avocado mixture onto salad plates.
9. Top with the salmon fillets and jalapeños.

CHAPTER FIVE

SOUP RECIPES

MINESTRONE SOUP

Yields: 8 servings
Serving Size: 1 bowl
Preparation Time: 15 minutes
Cooking Time: 1 hour and 10 minutes
Total Time: 1 hour and 25 minutes

INGREDIENTS

- ¼ tsp. fine sea salt
- 2 tbsp. olive oil
- 1 cup cooked chickpeas, drained
- 15 oz. can white beans, rinsed and drained
- 1 cup cabbage, sliced
- 2 stalks of celery, sliced
- 1 onion, chopped
- 4 cloves garlic, crushed and minced
- 6 cups reduced sodium vegetable broth
- 1 tbsp. fresh basil, chopped
- ¼ tsp. freshly ground black pepper
- ¾ cup Parmesan cheese, grated
- ¼ cup fresh parsley, chopped
- 28 oz. canned tomatoes, undrained
- ¼ cup tomato paste
- 1 bay leaf
- 1 cup dried fusilli pasta
- 2 carrots, chopped

COOKING INSTRUCTIONS

1. Put the olive oil in a soup pot on medium heat.
2. Sauté the onion and garlic for 6 minutes.
3. Then add the stock, basil, parsley, carrots, cabbage, celery, tomatoes, tomato paste and bay leaf.
4. Then stay for 40 minutes.
5. Add the pasta, chickpeas and white beans into it.
6. Simmer for 20 minutes.
7. Season with the salt and pepper.
8. Garnish on the top from cheese before serving.

MEATBALL NOODLE SOUP

Yields: 4 servings
Serving Size: 1 bowl
Preparation Time: 10 minutes
Cooking Time: 20 minutes
Total Time: 30 minutes

INGREDIENTS

- 1 cup green cabbage, shredded
- 1 lb. sausage, casings removed
- 3 tbsp. white vinegar
- ¼ tsp. sea salt
- ¼ cup whole wheat breadcrumbs
- ½ cup carrots, shredded
- 4 green onions, sliced
- 1 tbsp. vegetable oil
- 8 cups reduced sodium chicken stock
- 8 oz. capellini pasta

- 1 tsp. sesame oil

COOKING INSTRUCTIONS

1. First mix the sausage and breadcrumbs in a bowl.
2. Mode meatballs from the mixture.
3. Pour the oil in a soup pot on medium heat.
4. Cook the meatballs for 8 to 10 minutes.
5. Then pour in the stock and bring to a boil.
6. Add the capellini pasta.
7. Cook until the pasta is firm but not mushy.
8. In a bowl, combine the sesame oil, vinegar and salt.
9. Add the rest of the ingredients to the pot.
10. And cook until the carrots are soft but still firm.
11. Then serve in bowls.

RED LENTIL SOUP

Yields: 6 servings
Serving Size: 1 bowl
Preparation Time: 10 minutes
Cooking Time: 25 minutes
Total Time: 35 minutes

INGREDIENTS

- 1 tsp. ground cumin
- 1 carrot, diced
- 2 tbsp. tomato paste
- 1 onion, diced
- ¾ tsp. fine sea salt
- 1 tsp. mint, chopped
- 4 cloves garlic, crushed and minced

- 7 cups reduced sodium vegetable stock
- 1 ¼ cup red lentils, rinsed and drained

COOKING INSTRUCTIONS

1. Put the onion, garlic, stock, lentils, carrot, cumin and tomato paste in a soup pot. Mix well.
2. Bring to a boil, and then simmer for 25 minutes.
3. Alienate contents to an immersion blender.
4. Blend until becomes creamy.
5. Season with the salt and garnish with the mint before serving.

MEXICAN CHICKEN SOUP

Yields: 4 servings
Serving Size: 1 bowl
Preparation Time: 15 minutes
Cooking Time: 20 minutes
Total Time: 35 minutes

INGREDIENTS

- 1 clove garlic, mashed
- 1 cup hot water
- 2 dried ancho chilies, stems removed
- 1 qt. reduced sodium chicken broth
- 2 carrots, chopped
- 8 tortilla chips, crushed
- 4 tsp. feta cheese, crumbled
- ¼ cup avocado, diced
- ½ lb. chicken breasts (boneless and skinless), sliced into strips

- ½ tsp. fine sea salt
- ¼ tsp. ground black pepper
- 14.5oz. unsalted canned diced tomatoes, undrained
- Lime wedges
- 1 tsp. fresh cilantro, chopped

COOKING INSTRUCTIONS

1. Pour the water into a glass bowl.
2. Soak the chilies in it for 10 minutes.
3. Then put the chilies and water in a blender.
4. Pulse to purée.
5. In a soup pot, add the stock, garlic, tomatoes, and carrots.
6. Add the chili purée.
7. Simmer for 20 minutes.
8. Add the chicken and simmer until fully cooked.
9. Season the soup with the salt and pepper.
10. Serve with the lime wedges, cilantro, feta cheese, avocado and tortilla chips.

ROASTED BUTTERNUT SQUASH WITH CARDAMOM SOUP

Yields: 12 servings
Serving Size: 1 bowl
Preparation Time: 20 minutes
Cooking Time: 50 minutes
Total Time: 1 hour and 10 minutes

INGREDIENTS

- ½ tsp. freshly ground black pepper
- 1 ¼ tsp. ground cardamom

- 3 tbsp. olive oil
- ¾ tsp. fine sea salt, divided
- 2 onions, chopped
- ½ cup heavy cream, divided
- 12 cups butternut squash cubes
- ½ cup dry white wine
- 6 cups reduced sodium vegetable stock
- 1 tbsp. fresh thyme, chopped

COOKING INSTRUCTIONS

1. Preheat your oven to 425*F.
2. Place the onions, thyme and butternut squash in a large baking pan.
3. Toss in the oil and season with half of the salt and pepper.
4. Roast for 20 minutes.
5. Then put the roasted vegetables in a large soup pot.
6. Add the cardamom, wine and vegetable stock.
7. Stay for 10 minutes.
8. Purée the contents using an immersion blender.
9. Season with the remaining salt and pepper.
10. And reheat before serving.

CREAMY CAULIFLOWER & BROCCOLI SOUP

Yields: 4 servings
Serving Size: 1 bowl
Preparation Time: 10 minutes
Cooking Time: 40 minutes
Total Time: 50 minutes

INGREDIENTS

- 1 cup sourdough bread cubes
- 2 cups cauliflower florets, chopped
- 6 cups reduced sodium vegetable stock
- 1 potato, sliced into cubes
- 1 tbsp. olive oil
- 2 cups broccoli florets, chopped
- ¾ tsp. fine sea salt
- ½ onion, chopped

COOKING INSTRUCTIONS

1. Put the oil in a soup pot on medium heat.
2. Put the onion and cook until soft and translucent.
3. Add the potato and bread cubes and cook for 6 to 7 minutes.
4. Pour in the stock.
5. Add the cauliflower and broccoli into it.
6. Season with salt.
7. Simmer for 30 minutes.
8. Purée the contents in an immersion blender.
9. And reheat before serving.

TOMATO BULGUR SOUP

Yields: 4 servings
Serving Size: 1 bowl
Preparation Time: 10 minutes
Cooking Time: 30 minutes
Total Time: 40 minutes

INGREDIENTS

- ½ tsp. ground cinnamon
- 1 tsp. ground coriander
- 4 cups reduced sodium vegetable stock, divided
- 1 tbsp. freshly squeezed lemon juice
- 14 oz. unsalted canned diced tomatoes
- 1 cup bulgur wheat, uncooked
- 2 tbsp. fresh parsley leaves, chopped
- 1 clove garlic, crushed and minced
- 1 onion, minced

COOKING INSTRUCTIONS

1. Put two cups of the vegetable stock in a soup pot.
2. Boil for 10 minutes.
3. Add the garlic and onion and simmer for 5 minutes.
4. Add the cinnamon and coriander and cook for 1 minute.
5. Then add the bulgur and cook for half a minute.
6. Make sure to stir frequently.
7. Pour the remaining stock along with the tomatoes and their juices.
8. Bring to a boil and then simmer for 10 minutes.
9. Mix in the lemon juice.
10. Garnish with the parsley before serving.

BEET SOUP

Yields: 4 servings
Serving Size: 1 bowl
Preparation Time: 15 minutes
Cooking Time: 2 hours

Total Time: 2 hours and 15 minutes

63

INGREDIENTS

- 1 onion, chopped
- ½ tsp. fine sea salt
- 6 beets, scrubbed, rinsed and divided
- 1 tbsp. fresh chives, chopped
- ½ tsp. sugar
- 1 tbsp. red wine vinegar
- 1 tbsp. fresh dill, chopped
- 6 cups reduced sodium vegetable stock
- 2 tsp. caraway seeds

COOKING INSTRUCTIONS

1. Preheat your oven up to 400*F.
2. Coat the three beets with foil.
3. Then put on a baking pan.
4. And bake for 1 hour.
5. Remove the foil and slice thinly.
6. Chop the remaining beets.
7. Put in a saucepan over medium heat along with the stock, caraway seeds and onion.
8. Bring to a boil and then simmer for 50 minutes.
9. Strain out the solids.
10. Then put the liquid back in the pan.
11. Add the salt, sugar and vinegar to the roasted beets
12. Garnish with chives and dill before serving.

CHAPTER SIX

PORK RECIPES

GRILLED PORK WITH CHIMICCHURI

Yields: 4 servings
Serving Size: 1 pork chop
Preparation Time: 15 minutes
Cooking Time: 20 minutes
Total Time: 35 minutes

INGREDIENTS

- 1 cup parsley
- 4 pork chops
- ½ tsp. coarse sea salt
- ½ tsp. freshly cracked black pepper
- 1 tbsp. water
- 1 tsp. olive oil
- 3 tbsp. olive oil
- 2 tbsp. white onion, chopped
- 2 cloves garlic, crushed and minced
- ½ cup cilantro
- 2 tbsp. red wine vinegar
- ½ tsp. red chili pepper, crushed
- ½ tsp. fine sea salt

COOKING INSTRUCTIONS

1. Take the first nine ingredients in a blender or food processor and blend it well.
2. Then return all the mixture in a bowl.

3. First preheat the grill.
4. Brush the pork chops with the remaining oil.
5. Sprinkle the coarse salt and pepper onto the chops.
6. Roast until it fully cooked from both sides.
7. Plate up it with the chimichurri sauce.

CARIBBEAN PORK TENDERLOIN

Yields: 6 servings
Serving Size: 1 pork slice
Preparation Time: 15 minutes
Cooking Time: 20 minutes
Total Time: 35 minutes

INGREDIENTS

- 2 tsp. vegetable oil
- ¾ tsp. nutmeg, grated
- 2 bananas, peeled and sliced thickly
- 3 green onions, sliced thinly
- 1 cup freshly squeezed orange juice
- 1 clove garlic, chopped
- 1 lb. pork tenderloins
- 3 tbsp. lime juice
- 8 pineapple rings
- ¼ cup vinegar
- ¼ cup tamari
- ¾ tsp. ground cinnamon
- 2 tsp. ground allspice
- 1 Serrano chili, seeded and minced

COOKING INSTRUCTIONS

1. Add the vinegar, green onion, orange juice, lime juice, tamari, nutmeg, ground cinnamon, allspice, Serrano chili and garlic all together in a dish. Mix it well.
2. Give coat to the pork with this mixture.
3. And refrigerate it for 4 hours.
4. Grease your grill and preheat it to a medium setting.
5. Then grill the pork for about 15 minutes, turning it to cook evenly from all sides.
6. Sprinkle the oil onto the bananas.
7. Also grill the bananas and pineapple.
8. Serve the grilled pork and garnish it with the fruits.

PORK STIR FRY

Yields: 4 servings
Serving Size: 1 cup
Preparation Time: 15 minutes
Cooking Time: 15 minutes
Total Time: 30 minutes

INGREDIENTS

- 1 lb. pork cutlets, sliced into strips
- 1 tsp. fish sauce
- 2 limes, quarter cut
- ¼ tsp. sea salt
- ¼ tsp. black pepper
- 1 bunch scallions, sliced
- ¼ lb. mushrooms
- 1 tbsp. vegetable oil
- 1-inch ginger root, peeled and chopped

- 1 clove garlic, chopped
- 1 cup snow peas, strings removed
- 1 cup cilantro leaves
- 1 red bell pepper, sliced
- 1 yellow bell pepper, sliced
- 8 oz. canned water chestnuts, rinsed and cut into half
- 1 cup shredded cabbage
- 1 tbsp. rice vinegar
- 1 tbsp. shoyu sauce
- ½ tsp. hot chili sauce

COOKING INSTRUCTIONS

1. First rub the pork strips with the salt and pepper.
2. Take a large skillet on high heat.
3. Add the oil and cook the pork strips in it for 4 minutes.
4. Return them in a bowl. Keep it warm.
5. Add unto it, the ginger, garlic and scallion to the skillet and cook for 1 minute.
6. Then put on the mushrooms and cook for 3 minutes.
7. Add in the bell peppers and let it cook for 5 minutes.
8. Throw it in the water chestnuts and cabbage and cook until wilted (fade away).
9. Return the pork strips back to the skillet.
10. Add into it the rest of the ingredients except for the last two.
11. At the end garnish it with the cilantro and lime before platter.

FETTUCCINE WITH PORK MOLE

Yields: 4 servings

Serving Size: 1 bowl

Preparation Time: 15 minutes

Cooking Time: 30 minutes

Total Time: 45 minutes

INGREDIENTS

1. ½ tsp. ground cloves
2. ½ tsp. nutmeg, grated
3. 2 tbsp. olive oil, divided
4. 1 tsp. dried oregano
5. 1 tsp. ground cumin
6. 1 lb. pork, cut into cubes
7. 10 oz. fettuccine, cooked according to package directions
8. 1 onion, chopped
9. 28 oz. canned diced tomatoes, undrained
10. 1 tsp. chili garlic sauce
11. ⅔ cup seedless raisins
12. ½ cup reduced sodium chicken stock
13. ¼ cup almonds, sliced
14. 4 tsp. cocoa powder
15. ½ tsp. ground cinnamon
16. Salt to taste

COOKING INSTRUCTIONS

1. Pour 1 tablespoon of the oil in a skillet on medium heat.
2. Brown the pork from all sides. Push it to one side.
3. Pour the remaining oil into it.
4. Sauté the onions for 5 minutes.
5. Transfer the onions and the rest of the ingredients (except the fettuccine) to a blender.
6. Blend until it becomes smooth.
7. Simmer for 20 minutes.
8. Mix the pasta in the sauce and top with the pork.

PORK CHOPS WITH SHALLOTS & APPLE SLICES

Yields: 4 servings
Serving Size: 1 pork chop
Preparation Time: 10 minutes
Cooking Time: 21 minutes
Total Time: 31 minutes

INGREDIENTS

- 4 pork loin chops with bone
- ½ cup barbecue sauce, divided
- 3 shallots, sliced thinly
- Salt and pepper to taste
- Cooking spray
- 1 apple, cut into halves, core removed and sliced thinly
- 2 tbsp. olive oil

COOKING INSTRUCTIONS

1. Preheat your oven to 450*F.
2. Brush the baking pan with cooking spray.
3. Arrange the apple and shallots on the pan properly.
4. Shower the salt and pepper on the top.
5. Pour the oil onto a skillet on medium heat.
6. Rub the salt and pepper onto the pork chops.
7. And cook for 3 minutes per side.
8. Then place the pork chops on the baking pan.
9. Cover it with the barbecue sauce.
10. Lower the temperature to 375 *F and bake for about 15 minutes.

PORK WITH RASPBERRY SAUCE

Yields: 4 servings
Serving Size: 2 pork tenderloin slices
Preparation Time: 10 minutes
Cooking Time: 20 minutes
Total Time: 30 minutes

INGREDIENTS

- ¼ tsp. sea salt
- ¼ tsp. black pepper
- 1 tsp. cornstarch mixed with 1 tbsp. water
- 2 tsp. honey mustard
- 1 lb. pork tenderloin, sliced into 8 pieces
- 16 oz. fresh raspberries
- 1 tbsp. olive oil
- 2 shallots, chopped
- ½ cup dry white wine
- 1 cup reduced sodium beef stock

COOKING INSTRUCTIONS

1. Season the pork with the salt and pepper.
2. Take a skillet and put it on medium heat.
3. Pour the oil and wait until it becomes hot.
4. Add the pork slices and cook for 4 minutes each side.
5. Then transfer it to a plate.
6. Put the shallots in the skillet and cook for about half a minute.
7. Add the wine and stock in it.
8. Scrape the brown bits using a wooden spoon.
9. Add the stock and boil for 5 minutes
10. Then stir in the cornstarch mixture.
11. Let it cook for addition minute.
12. Add the raspberries and mustard, then cook it for 2 more minutes.

13. Drizzle the sauce over the pork slices and serve while warm.

GRILLED PORK & VEGETABLE PINWHEEL

Yields: 6 servings
Serving Size: 2 slices
Preparation Time: 10 minutes
Cooking Time: 25 minutes
Total Time: 35 minutes

INGREDIENTS

- 1 red bell pepper, chopped
- ½ tsp. ground cumin
- 3 cloves garlic, chopped
- 1 ½ lb. pork tenderloins, trimmed and butterfly-cut
- 1 ½ tsp. paprika
- 1 ½ tsp. chili powder
- ⅛ tsp. cayenne pepper
- 1 tsp. fine sea salt, divided
- ¼ tsp. black pepper
- 1 tbsp. olive oil
- 1 onion, chopped
- 1 lb. mushrooms, chopped

COOKING INSTRUCTIONS

1. Combine the cumin, paprika, chili powder, cayenne, and half of the salt in a bowl.
2. Pour the oil into a skillet on medium heat.
3. Then sauté the onion, red bell pepper and mushrooms for 7 minutes.
4. And add the garlic and cook for 1 minute.

5. Season with the remaining salt.
6. First preheat your grill.
7. Season the pork with the spicy mixture.
8. And stuff each one with the vegetable mixture.
9. Then roll and secure with twine.
10. Grill it for 12 - 15 minutes.
11. Let it cool before slicing and serving.

SHREDDED PORK WITH ONION RINGS

Yields: 8 servings
Serving Size: 1 cup
Preparation Time: 20 minutes
Cooking Time: 1 hour and 8 minutes
Total Time: 1 hour and 28 minutes

INGREDIENTS

- 2 cups freshly squeezed orange juice
- ¼ tsp. dried oregano
- ½ cup white wine vinegar, divided
- ½ white onion, sliced into rings
- 3 lb. pork butt, trimmed and sliced into cubes
- 1 tbsp. vegetable oil
- ½ white onion, sliced
- 2 cloves garlic, minced
- 1 tsp. sea salt
- ½ tsp. black pepper
- 2 bay leaves
- 1 tbsp. lime juice

COOKING INSTRUCTIONS

1. First apply the salt and pepper onto the pork.
2. Then sprinkle the oil into a pot and set it over high heat.
3. Brown the pork for about 2 minutes on each side.
4. Then transfer into a plate.
5. Then lower the heat and cook the white onions for 4 minutes.
6. Add the garlic and bay leaves into it and cook for 2 minutes.
7. Put down the pork back into the pot.
8. Muddle the lime juice, orange juice, and half of the vinegar.
9. Simmer (boil) it for 1 hour.
10. Remove the pork and shred (pieces) using two forks.
11. Mingle the onion rings with the remaining vinegar and oregano.
12. Then dish up the shredded pork with the onion rings.

PORK & BACON TENDERLOIN

Yields: 6 servings
Serving Size: 2 slices
Preparation Time: 10 minutes
Cooking Time: 35 minutes
Total Time: 45 minutes

INGREDIENTS

- 1 fennel bulb, cut into half and sliced
- 6 slices bacon
- 1 tbsp. fresh rosemary leaves, chopped
- 2 ½ tsp. fennel seeds, crushed
- 4 cloves garlic, chopped
- ¼ tsp. red chili flakes, crushed
- ¾ tsp. sea salt
- 2 tbsp. lemon zest

- ¼ tsp. ground black pepper
- 2 tsp. plus 1 tbsp. lemon juice, divided
- 3 tsp. olive oil, divided
- 1 ½ lb. pork tenderloin

COOKING INSTRUCTIONS

1. Preheat your oven up to 425*F.
2. In a mixing bowl, add the garlic, rosemary, lemon zest, fennel seeds, red chili flakes, salt and pepper together and mix it well.
3. Add half of the oil and 2 teaspoons of lemon juice in it.
4. Rub this mixture all over on the pork.
5. Then in a baking pan, spread the fennel and sprinkle with the remaining oil and lemon juice.
6. Wrap the bacon around the pork tenderloin and place this on the baking pan.
7. And roast the pork at 145*F for 35 minutes.
8. Let it sit for 10 minutes before slicing into 12 portions.

PORK WITH APPLES & FENNEL

Yields: 6 servings
Serving Size: 1 cup
Preparation Time: 15 minutes
Cooking Time: 1 hour
Total Time: 1 hour and 15 minutes

INGREDIENTS

- 1 cup dried apples, sliced
- 14 dried prunes, sliced
- 5 apples, peeled, core removed and sliced into cubes

- 3 sprigs parsley
- Salt and pepper to taste
- 1 ½ lb. pork butt, sliced into cubes
- 2 tbsp. vegetable oil
- 1 fennel bulb, core removed and diced
- 1 onion, diced
- 1 cup dry white wine
- 2 cups reduced sodium chicken stock
- 6 fresh sage leaves, sliced
- ½ cup apple juice
- 1 bay leaf

COOKING INSTRUCTIONS

1. Sprinkle (spread) the salt and pepper onto the pork cubes.
2. Then splash oil into a pot.
3. And cook the pork in the oil until it becomes brown.
4. Detach the pork and place it on a plate.
5. Add the fennel and onion to the pot and sauté them for 10 minutes.
6. Take some white wine and simmer (boil) it for 5 minutes.
7. Return the pork to the pot.
8. Add the rest of the ingredients into it and cook for 1 hour.

CHAPTER SEVEN

BEEF/LAMB RECIPES

MEAT BAGEL

INGREDIENTS

- 2 pounds of ground pork
- 2 large eggs
- Butter/grass fed ghee/bacon fat etc.
- 2/3 cup tomato sauce
- 1 tablespoon salt
- ½ tablespoon pepper
- 1 tablespoon
- Paprika
- 1 ½ onions, finely diced

COOKING INSTRUCTIONS

1. Preheat the oven to 400F.
2. Line a baking dish with parchment paper.
3. Sauté the onions until translucent over medium heat with some cooking fat, like butter, grass fed ghee etc.
4. When the onions is cool add them to the meat.
5. Add all the ingredients together including the cooked onions in a bowl and mix.
6. Mix well enough to evenly distribute the spices.

7. Then divide the meat into 6 portions. Use your hands to roll a portion into a ball and then indent the middle, and flatten slightly to form the appearance of a bagel.
8. Place the bagel looking meat in the dish and repeat with each of the portions of meat.
9. Bake for 40 minutes or until the meat is fully cooked.
10. Allow the meat bagels to cool. Slice the meat bagel just like a regular bagel.
11. Fill the meat bagel with topping such as tomato slices, lettuce, onions etc.
12. You can enjoy now.

BEEF KEBAB

Yields: 4 servings
Serving Size: 1 skewer
Preparation Time: 20 minutes
Cooking Time: 20 minutes
Total Time: 40 minutes

INGREDIENTS

- ½ tsp. fine sea salt
- ¼ tsp. black pepper
- 1 tsp. olive oil ½ tsp. ground allspice
- ⅛ tsp. cayenne pepper
- 1 ¼ lb. lean ground beef
- 3 tbsp. parsley, chopped
- ½ tsp. ground cinnamon

COOKING INSTRUCTIONS

1. First preheat your grill.
2. Then in a bowl, mix all the ingredients except the oil.
3. Then make small balls from the beef mixture.
4. Then include this in a metal skewers.
5. Brush the grill with oil.

6. Grill until fully cooked from all sides.

SLOPPY JOES

Yields: 4 servings
Serving Size: 1 bun
Preparation Time: 15 minutes
Cooking Time: 15 minutes
Total Time: 30 minutes

INGREDIENTS

- 4 hamburger buns, toasted
- 1 onion, chopped
- 2 tbsp. cider vinegar
- 1 tbsp. brown sugar
- Black pepper to taste
- 1 red bell pepper, chopped
- 1 tbsp. olive oil
- 2 cloves garlic, chopped
- 1 ¼ lb. lean ground beef
- 2 cups tomato-based pasta sauce
- 1 ½ tbsp. Worcestershire sauce

COOKING INSTRUCTIONS

1. First pour the oil into a skillet on medium heat.
2. Sauté the onion until it becomes soft.
3. Add the bell pepper into it and cook for 5 minutes.
4. Then add the garlic and cook for 1 minute.
5. Also add the beef and cook until becomes brown.

6. Stir in the rest of the ingredients, except from the buns.
7. Boil and then simmer for about 5 minutes.
8. Place the mixture onto the burger buns and serve it.

BEEF TACO PIZZA

Yields: 6 servings
Serving Size: 1 slice
Preparation Time: 10 minutes
Cooking Time: 30 minutes
Total Time: 40 minutes

INGREDIENTS

- ¾ cup pinto beans, rinsed and drained
- 1 lb. whole wheat pizza dough
- ¾ cup corn kernels
- Cooking spray
- ¼ cup salsa
- ½ lb. ground beef
- ¼ cup cheddar cheese, shredded
- 1 tbsp. chili powder

COOKING INSTRUCTIONS

1. First preheat your oven to 450*F.
2. Then take a pan and brown the beef in it for about 7 minutes.
3. Add the chili powder and corn into it.
4. Stir it in the beans.
5. And cook for a few more minutes.
6. Then press the pizza dough into a pizza pan.

7. Spread the beef mixture on the top of the dough and make a proper layer of it.
8. Then add on the top of beef chopped cheese.
9. Bake it for 20 minutes.
10. After baking remove the pizza from oven and serve it.

CAJUN BEEF

Yields: 4 servings
Serving Size: 1 cup
Preparation Time: 10 minutes
Cooking Time: 20 minutes
Total Time: 30 minutes

INGREDIENTS

- 15 oz. unsalted kidney beans, rinsed and drained
- 1 cup onion, chopped
- 20 oz. brown rice, cooked according to package directions
- 1 cup celery, sliced
- 1 red bell pepper, sliced
- 1 jalapeño pepper, chopped
- ¾ lb. lean ground beef
- 4 tsp. low sodium Cajun seasoning, divided
- ½ cup reduced sodium vegetable stock
- ¼ cup parsley, chopped

COOKING INSTRUCTIONS

1. Take the beef and season it with half of the Cajun powder.
2. Then brown the beef in a pan for 10 minutes.
3. Add the celery, onion, pepper and jalapeño in the pan.
4. Season it with the rest of the Cajun powder.

5. Then cook it for 8 minutes.
6. Add the broth into it.
7. Cook for 2 to 3 minutes more.
8. Add the parsley and stir very well.
9. Spoon the mixture on top of the rice before serving.

PASTA SHELLS STUFFED WITH BEEF & SPINACH

Yields: 6 servings
Serving Size: 1 bowl
Preparation Time: 15 minutes
Cooking Time: 45 minutes
Total Time: 1 hour

INGREDIENTS

- 16 oz. spinach, chopped
- 15 oz. marinara sauce
- 1 ¼ cup ricotta cheese
- 8 oz. jumbo pasta shells, cooked according to package directions
- ¾ lb. lean ground beef
- 1 ¼ cup mozzarella cheese, shredded

COOKING INSTRUCTIONS

1. First preheat your oven to 350*F.
2. Then put your skillet on medium heat.
3. Brown the beef for 5 - 7 minutes in the pan.
4. Then drain the fat from it.
5. In a bowl, mix the beef with cheese and spinach.
6. Pour half of the marinara sauce on a baking pan.

7. Stuff the pasta shells with the beef mixture and put them on top of the marinara sauce.
8. Pour the remaining marinara on top of the pasta shells.
9. Take some of chopped cheese on top of it.
10. Then bake it in the oven for 35 minutes.
11. After baking remove it from the oven and serve it warm.

COUSCOUS & BEEF LETTUCE WRAP

Yields: 6 servings
Serving Size: 1 lettuce wrap
Preparation Time: 15 minutes
Cooking Time: 15 minutes
Total Time: 30 minutes

INGREDIENTS

- 1 cup cucumber, sliced
- 1 cup cabbage, sliced
- 1 cup carrot, sliced
- ½ cup mint, chopped 1 ¼ cups water
- 1 lb. ground beef
- ¼ cup organic steak sauce
- 6 oz. organic couscous
- 1 head iceberg lettuce, core removed
- 1 cup green onion, sliced

COOKING INSTRUCTIONS

1. First brown the beef in a skillet on medium heat for 5 minutes.

2. Add the steak sauce and cook for 7 minutes.
3. Add water and couscous into it and mix well.
4. Bring it to a boil.
5. Simmer (stay) it for 7 minutes.
6. Fluff the couscous using a fork.
7. Then insert a spoonful of beef mixture onto the lettuce leaf.
8. Wrap and secure it with a toothpick.
9. Repeat the same procedure for the rest of the ingredients.

BEEF EMPANADA

Yields: 8 servings
Serving Size: 2 empanadas
Preparation Time: 20 minutes
Cooking Time: 40 minutes
Total Time: 1 hour

INGREDIENTS

- ½ cup butter, cut into small pieces
- 14 oz. canned diced tomatoes
- 4 eggs, hardboiled and quarter cut
- 2 egg yolks, divided
- ½ cup water
- 1 tbsp. vegetable oil
- 1 tsp. fine sea salt
- 2 ½ cups all-purpose flour
- 1 onion, chopped
- ½ cup Kalamata olives, chopped
- 1 lb. ground beef

COOKING INSTRUCTIONS

1. First mix the salt and flour in a bowl and mix it well.
2. Then fold it in the butter. And mix well.
3. In another bowl, combine one egg yolk with water.
4. Mix all these ingredients very well.
5. Dust the working surface with flour.
6. Knead (mix the dough through hands) until it becomes smooth.
7. Wrap with cling wrap (string)) and refrigerate it for 1 hour.
8. Place the skillet over medium heat.
9. Pour some oil in it and sauté the onion for 7 minutes.
10. Then reduce the heat more and add the olives, beef and tomatoes.
11. And cook for more 12 minutes.
12. Preheat your oven to 425* F.
13. Make slices of the dough into sixteen equal portions.
14. Roll out the dough to create a small circle.
15. Place a scoop of the beef mixture in the middle of the circle.
16. Add a quarter of the hardboiled egg and fill it properly.
17. Brush the edges with the water and egg mixture.
18. Fold and press to seal.
19. Repeat the same recipe for the rest of the round sheets.
20. Brush all surfaces of the empanadas with the egg and water mixture.
21. Arrange the empanadas in a baking pan and bake it in the oven for 30 minutes.

BEEF & BEAN CHILI

Yields: 4 servings
Serving Size: 1 bowl
Preparation Time: 10 minutes
Cooking Time: 35 minutes
Total Time: 45 minutes

INGREDIENTS

- 1 tsp. ground cumin
- 1 lb. lean ground beef
- 2 tbsp. olive oil
- 2 tsp. dried oregano
- ½ cup fresh cilantro, chopped
- ½ tsp. red chili flakes, crushed
- 2 tbsp. chili powder
- 15 oz. tomato sauce
- 1 onion, chopped
- 2 cloves garlic, crushed and minced
- 1 cup water
- 1 cup kidney beans, cooked
- 1 cup black beans, cooked
- Salt to taste

COOKING INSTRUCTIONS

1. Take the olive oil in a soup pot on medium heat.
2. Then sauté the onion and garlic in oil for 5 minutes.
3. Add the oregano, chili flakes, chili powder, and cumin into the oil.
4. Cook for an additional minute.
5. Then add the ground beef and cook it until it becomes brown.
6. Stir it in the tomato sauce, water and beans.
7. Season it with the salt.
8. Then bring it to a boil.
9. Boil it for 30 minutes.
10. Mingle it in the cilantro before serving.

MEXICAN BEEF

Yields: 4 servings
Serving Size: 1 bowl
Preparation Time: 15 minutes
Cooking Time: 27 minutes
Total Time: 42 minutes

INGREDIENTS

- 1 cup salsa
- 15 oz. black beans
- 2 cups reduced sodium chicken stock
- 1 cup corn kernels
- 2 cloves garlic, chopped
- 1 onion, chopped
- 2 tbsp. taco seasoning
- ½ lb. lean ground beef
- 1 zucchini, cut into cubes
- 15 oz. diced tomatoes

COOKING INSTRUCTIONS

1. Take the beef in a soup pot on medium heat.
2. Cook it until it becomes brown.
3. Then remove the beef and drain the fat. Then set aside.
4. Take garlic and onion in the same pot and cook for 7 minutes.
5. Season it with the taco mixture.
6. And add the rest of the ingredients into it.
7. Stay for 20 minutes.
8. Ladle (pour) into a soup bowl and serve warm.

BULGUR BEEF BURGER

Yields: 6 servings
Serving Size: 1 burger
Preparation Time: 20 minutes
Cooking Time: 20 minutes
Total Time: 40 minutes

INGREDIENTS

- 1 ¼ lb. lean ground beef
- ¾ cup onion, chopped
- 3 cups Romaine lettuce, chopped
- 2 tomatoes, sliced
- 2 cups water
- 1 cup bulgur wheat
- Cooking spray
- ½ cup parsley, chopped
- 6 whole wheat hamburger buns, toasted
- ½ tsp. ground allspice
- ½ tsp. ground cinnamon
- 1 tsp. ground cumin
- Salt and pepper to taste

COOKING INSTRUCTIONS

1. Boil water in a pot.
2. Add the bulgur wheat and simmer for 10 minutes.
3. Then remove from the stove.
4. Let sit for 5 minutes before fluffing with fork.
5. Grease and preheat your grill.
6. Get a bowl, combine the beef, bulgur, onion, parsley and spices.
7. Season with the salt and pepper.

8. Form 6 patties from the mixture.
9. Put the burger in the buns and add the lettuce and tomatoes before serving.

CHAPTER EIGHT

SNACK/DESSERT RECIPES

CINNAMON & APPLE OAT SQUARES

Yields: 16 servings
Serving Size: 1 square
Preparation Time: 15 minutes
Cooking Time: 1 hour
Total Time: 1 hour and 15 minutes

INGREDIENTS

- 2 cups unsweetened almond milk
- 2 tsp. pure vanilla extract
- ½ cup ground flax seeds
- 1 lb. apples, peeled, cored and grated
- Cooking spray
- ½ cup raisins
- 1 ½ cup oats
- ½ cup pecans, chopped
- 1 ½ tsp. ground cinnamon

COOKING INSTRUCTIONS

1. First preheat your oven to 350*F.
2. Take all the ingredients in a large mixing bowl.
3. Mix it well.
4. Then transfer mixture to a baking pan, coated with cooking spray.
5. Press and spread the mixture properly.

6. And bake for 1 hour.
7. Let it cool.
8. Then cut into 16 square shapes.

DATE & ALMOND BITES

Yields: 5 servings
Serving Size: 6 pieces
Preparation Time: 20 minutes
Cooking Time: 0 minutes
Total Time: 20 minutes

INGREDIENTS

- ¼ tsp. nutmeg, grated
- 1 tsp. pure almond extract
- Water
- ½ cup unsweetened almond butter
- 1 ¼ cup dates, pitted and chopped
- 1 ¼ cup rolled oats
- 1 tbsp. poppy seeds

COOKING INSTRUCTIONS

1. Take all the ingredients in a blender
2. Blend it until becomes smooth.
3. Sprinkle the mixture with a little bit of water.
4. Then make 30 balls of it.
5. Make it chill for a few hours before serving.

PLUM CRUMBLE

Yields: 8 servings
Serving Size: 1 slice
Preparation Time: 15 minutes
Cooking Time: 45 minutes
Total Time: 1 hour

INGREDIENTS

- 20 vanilla wafer cookies
- 1 cup almonds, sliced
- 1 ½ lb. plums, pitted and chopped
- 4 tbsp. butter, cut into cubes
- 1 tsp. ground cinnamon

COOKING INSTRUCTIONS

1. First preheat your oven to 350*F.
2. Take almonds in a food processor and blend it well.
3. Put the butter, cookies and cinnamon in a bowl.
4. Blend well.
5. Slowly add the mixture in the almonds and mix together.
6. Then arrange a layer of the plums on a baking pan.
7. Spread a layer of the almond mixture on the upper of the plums.
8. And bake for 45 minutes.
9. Let it cool then make slices of it and serve

GRANOLA COCONUT BARS

Yields: 12 servings
Serving Size: 1 bar
Preparation Time: 20 minutes
Cooking Time: 40 minutes
Total Time: 1 hour

INGREDIENTS

- 1 cup dried fruits, chopped
- 1 cup unsweetened coconut flakes
- ¼ cup honey
- 2 tsp. pure vanilla extract
- ¼ cup oat flour
- ½ cup pecans, chopped
- 1 ½ cup rolled oats
- ¾ cup unsweetened applesauce

COOKING INSTRUCTIONS

1. Preheat your oven to 350* F.
2. Line baking pan with parchment paper.
3. Then mix the coconut flakes and oats in a bowl.
4. And transfer to a baking sheet.
5. Bake for 10 minutes.
6. Let it cool.
7. In a large mixing bowl, combine the oat flour, pecans and dried fruits.
8. Mix it in the apple sauce.
9. And blend it well.
10. Then spread into an even layer on a baking pan.
11. And bake for 30 minutes.
12. Make slices of 12 bars.

LEMONADE WITH YOGURT

Yields: 6 servings
Serving Size: 1 glass
Preparation Time: 1 hour and 15 minutes
Cooking Time: 0 minutes
Total Time: 15 minutes

INGREDIENTS

- 1 cup strawberries, sliced
- 4 cups lemonade made with fresh lemons
- 2 tsp. honey
- 6 oz. plain yogurt
- 1 cup blackberries, sliced

COOKING INSTRUCTIONS

1. First pour the lemonade into a baking pan.
2. Put in the freezer for 1 hour.
3. Take it out and stir.
4. Then put it back until the lemonade is completely frozen.
5. Take a bowl, mix the honey and yogurt in it.
6. And beat with an electric mixer until you see soft peaks forming.
7. Take out the iced lemonade and scrape plight with wooden spoon.
8. Put the iced lemonade in serving cups and garnish with the berries and yogurt mixture.

SWEETENED BANANA POPS

Yields: 8 servings
Serving Size: 1 pop
Preparation Time: 15 minutes
Cooking Time: 0 minutes
Total Time: 15 minutes

INGREDIENTS

- 1 tsp. ground cinnamon
- ¼ cup brown sugar, divided
- 3 bananas
- 1 cup light sour cream

COOKING INSTRUCTIONS

1. Take 2 tablespoons brown sugar, the sour cream and the bananas in a food processor.
2. Pulse until becomes smooth.
3. Pour the mixture into popsicle molds.
4. Then put the remaining brown sugar and cinnamon in a bowl. Mix it well.
5. Sprinkle the sugar-cinnamon mixture onto the bananas mixture.
6. And freeze it for 8 hours.

BASIL & MANGO SORBET

Yields: 6 servings
Serving Size: 1 cup
Preparation Time: 15 minutes

Cooking Time: 0 minutes
Total Time: 15 minutes

INGREDIENTS

- 1 teaspoon lime zest
- 10 oz. mango, cut into cubes
- 1 cup unsweetened soy milk
- 2 tbsp. Thai basil leaves, chopped
- 1 tablespoon lime juice

COOKING INSTRUCTIONS

1. First put the mango in a food processor.
2. Add the basil, lime juice and lime zest in it.
3. Then pin the soymilk.
4. Pulse until becomes smooth.
5. Then divide the mixture among 6 cups.
6. Make it chill in the freezer for 30 minutes before serving.

BANANA & STRAWBERRY MILK SHAKE

Yields: 2 servings
Serving Size: 1 glass
Preparation Time: 10 minutes
Cooking Time: 0 minutes
Total Time: 10 minutes

INGREDIENTS

- 2 tbsp. almond butter
- 2 cups frozen banana
- ½ cup low fat milk

- 1 ½ cup strawberries, cut in half

COOKING INSTRUCTIONS

1. First blend banana, strawberries and milk until becomes smooth.
2. Then pour into 2 glasses.
3. Make a layer with the almond butter.
4. Make it chill in the refrigerator before serving.

DRIED FRUIT BITES

Yields: 2 servings
Serving Size: 1 cup
Preparation Time: 15 minutes
Cooking Time: 3 hours
Total Time: 3 hours and 15 minutes

INGREDIENTS

- 4 cups water
- ½ cup freshly squeezed lemon juice
- 1 ½ lb. nectarines, pitted and sliced

COOKING INSTRUCTIONS

1. First preheat your oven up to 200*F.
2. Mix the water and lemon juice in a bowl.
3. Then soak the nectarines in the lemon water for 10 minutes.
4. And arrange it on a baking pan.
5. Bake for 3 hours or until completely dried.

SPANISH CHICKPEAS

Yields: 2 servings
Serving Size: ½ bowl
Preparation Time: 2 minutes
Cooking Time: 30 minutes
Total Time: 32 minutes

INGREDIENTS

- 1 tsp. lemon juice
- 1 ½ tsp. smoked paprika
- 1 teaspoon lemon zest
- 15 oz. canned unsalted chickpeas, rinsed and drained

COOKING INSTRUCTIONS

1. First preheat your oven up to 350*F.
2. Toss all the ingredients in a bowl and mix well.
3. Then transfer to a baking pan.
4. And bake for 30 minutes.
5. Let it cool before serving.

APPLE SANDWICH

Yields: 2 servings
Serving Size: 1 sandwich
Preparation Time: 10 minutes
Cooking Time: 0 minutes
Total Time: 10 minutes

INGREDIENTS

- 3 tbsp. granola
- 2 apples, cut into thick rounds
- 1 tsp. lemon juice
- 3 tbsp. almond butter

COOKING INSTRUCTIONS

1. First brush the apple slices with lemon juice.
2. Then spread almond butter on top of it.
3. Then sprinkle with the granola.
4. And place the remaining apple slices on top.

CRISPY KALE CHIPS

Yields: 8 servings
Serving Size: 1 cup
Preparation Time: 10 minutes
Cooking Time: 45 minutes
Total Time: 55 minutes

INGREDIENTS

- 1 tbsp. onion powder
- ¼ cup unsweetened plain soy milk
- ¼ tsp. fine sea salt
- 2 bunches kale, torn into bite size pieces
- 1 cup red peppers, roasted and chopped
- 1 tablespoon lemon juice
- ¼ cup nutritional yeast

- 1 cup cashews
- 3 cloves garlic

COOKING INSTRUCTIONS

1. First soak the cashews in water for 1 hour.
2. Then preheat your oven to 275*F.
3. Take all the ingredients except the kale in a blender.
4. And blend until smooth.
5. Then cover baking pan with parchment.
6. Toss the kale with the cashew mixture.
7. Spread the kale in a single layer on a baking pan.
8. Bake it for 45 minutes.
9. Let it cool before serving.

SEASONED PUMPKIN SEEDS

Yields: 1 serving
Serving Size: 1 cup
Preparation Time: 5 minutes
Cooking Time: 10 minutes
Total Time: 15 minutes

INGREDIENTS

- 1 tbsp. reduced sodium vegetable broth
- 2 tbsp. nutritional yeast
- 1 cup pumpkin seeds
- 1 tbsp. parsley, chopped

COOKING INSTRUCTIONS

1. First preheat your oven up to 350*F.
2. Then put all the ingredients in a bowl.
3. And mix well.
4. Spread the mixture on a baking pan.
5. And bake for 10 minutes.

STONE FRUIT TRIFLE

Yields: 12 servings
Serving Size: 1 trifle dish
Preparation Time: 10 minutes
Cooking Time: 25 minutes
Total Time: 35 minutes

INGREDIENTS

- 2 cups low fat vanilla yogurt
- 2 tbsp. honey
- 3 lb. mixed stone fruits (plums, peaches, nectarines and so on), cut into halves and pitted
- 12 oz. gluten free angel food cake, sliced
- 1 tbsp. water
- 2 tbsp. fresh thyme leaves, chopped

COOKING INSTRUCTIONS

1. First preheat your grill.
2. In a bowl, mix together honey and water.
3. Coat the upper part of the fruits with a little bit of this mixture.
4. And grill for 10 minutes.

5. Flip and coat the other side as well.
6. Grill for another 10 minutes.
7. Next, grill the cake slices for 3 minutes.
8. Then cut the cake into bite size pieces.
9. Chop the grilled fruit into smaller pieces.
10. Mix with the thyme and remaining honey mixture.
11. Divide the yogurt into trifle dishes and top with this mixture.
12. Chill in the refrigerator for a few minutes before serving.

LEMON FLOATS

Yields: 4 servings
Serving Size: 1 glass
Preparation Time: 5 minutes
Cooking Time: 0 minutes
Total Time: 5 minutes

INGREDIENTS

- 8 sprigs rosemary, crushed
- 2 cups lemon gelato
- 1 lemon, seeded and quarter cut
- 2 tablespoons lemon juice

COOKING INSTRUCTIONS

1. Divide the gelato among 4 glasses.
2. Pour the lemon juice on the top of the gelato.
3. Garnish it with the rosemary and lemon wedges before serving.

CHAPTER NINE

POULTRY RECIPES

TURKEY WITH CORIANDER & PEPPERCORNS

Yields: 14 servings
Serving Size: 1 portion
Preparation Time: 20 minutes
Cooking Time: 3 hours
Total Time: 3 hours and 20 minutes

INGREDIENTS

- 3 tbsp. butter, softened
- 3 tbsp. coriander seeds
- 15 lb. turkey, giblets and neck removed
- 2 tsp. fennel seeds
- 1 tbsp. black peppercorns
- 1 ½ tbsp. pink peppercorns
- 4 bay leaves
- 6 tbsp. coarse sea salt
- ¼ cup grapefruit zest
- 3 tbsp. brown sugar

COOKING INSTRUCTIONS

1. Take the peppercorns, coriander, fennel and bay leaves in a skillet on medium heat.
2. Then cook it for 3 - 5 minutes.

3. Leave it cool in a bowl.
4. Use a grinder to beat the mixture and make it powder.
5. Add the zest, sugar, butter and salt. Mix it well.
6. Pour the mixture all over on the turkey.
7. Roast it in the oven at 325*F for 1 hour.
8. Then increase the temperature to 375*F and roast it for 2 more hours.
9. Then garnish it as you want and serve it to your friends and family.

CRISPY SKIN BAKED TURKEY

Yields: 14 servings
Serving Size: 1 portion
Preparation Time: 20 minutes
Cooking Time: 1 hour and 40 minutes
Total Time: 2 hours

INGREDIENTS

- ¼ cup olive oil
- 2 tbsp. fresh rosemary leaves, chopped
- 1 whole turkey, giblets removed
- Salt and pepper to taste

COOKING INSTRUCTIONS

1. First you have to dry the turkey using paper towels.
2. Place it in a roasting pan when it becomes roast then chill it in the refrigerator overnight.
3. The next day preheat your oven to 350* F.
4. In a bowl take the oil, rosemary, salt and pepper and mix it well.
5. Rub the mixture all over on the turkey.

6. Season the inside of the turkey as well.
7. Roast it in the oven for 1 hour and 15 minutes.
8. Then raise the temperature to 475* F and roast it for another 15 minutes.
9. Remove it from the oven.
10. Wait for about 25 minutes before slicing.
11. And then serve it.

CHICKEN TETRAZZINI

Yields: 6 servings
Serving Size: 1 cup
Preparation Time: 15 minutes
Cooking Time: 30 minutes
Total Time: 45 minutes

INGREDIENTS

- 1 tbsp. olive oil
- Cooking oil spray
- ½ tbsp. butter
- 8 oz. mushrooms, sliced
- Salt and pepper to taste
- 4 tbsp. chives, chopped and divided
- ½ lb. whole wheat angel hair noodles, cooked according to package directions
- 1 cup frozen peas, thawed
- 2 cups chicken breast meat, cooked and shredded
- 6 tbsp. Parmesan cheese, grated and divided
- ½ onion, minced
- 2 ½ tbsp. flour
- 1 cup reduced sodium chicken stock
- ¼ cup low fat milk
- ¼ tsp. ground nutmeg

1. First preheat your oven up to 375*F.
2. Coat casserole dish with the cooking spray.
3. Take a skillet on medium heat.
4. In that skillet sauté the onion in the butter.
5. Then add mushrooms, salt and pepper into it.
6. Cook it for a few minutes.
7. Add the peas into it and cook it for 2 more minutes.
8. Put the cooked pasta in a bowl and top with the onion mixture.
9. In the same saucepan heat the olive oil and add it in the flour and stock.
10. Mix it well until there are no more lumps in it.
11. Add the milk and nutmeg in the mixture.
12. Season the mixture with the salt and pepper.
13. Toss the pasta in the mixture.
14. On the top put the cheeses.
15. Bake for 15 minutes.
16. And serve it while warm.

CHICKEN WITH OLIVES & ROASTED RED PEPPER

Yields: 6 servings
Serving Size: 1 slice
Preparation Time: 15 minutes
Cooking Time: 15 minutes
Total Time: 30 minutes

INGREDIENTS

- 1 cup red peppers, roasted and sliced
- 2 tsp. dried tarragon
- 1 tsp. ground black pepper
- 2 cups chicken, cooked and shredded

- 1 sheet frozen puff pastry
- 1 egg, beaten
- ½ cup olives, chopped
- 1 cup Parmesan cheese, shredded

COOKING INSTRUCTIONS

1. First preheat your oven up to 400*F.
2. Then cut the pastry sheet into two long rectangular shapes.
3. Put these sheets in a baking pan.
4. (Fold) the borders of the pastry sheet.
5. Brush the sheets with the beaten egg (the eggs you have already beaten in a bowl)
6. Then take the peppers, chicken and olives and pour them inside the border.
7. Sprinkle the tarragon, pepper and cheese on top of the mixture.
8. Bake the mixture in the oven for 15 minutes.
9. After baking slice each sheet into 3 pieces.
10. Serve it while it is warm.

CHICKEN SONOMA

Yields: 8 servings
Serving Size: 1 cup
Preparation Time: 10 minutes
Cooking Time: 25 minutes
Total Time: 35 minutes

INGREDIENTS

- ¾ cup pecan pieces, toasted
- 2 tsp. poppy seeds
- 2 lb. chicken breasts (boneless and skinless)
- 5 tsp. honey

- 1 cup mayonnaise
- 4 tsp. apple cider vinegar
- ¼ tsp. fine sea salt
- ¼ tsp. ground black pepper
- ½ cup water
- 3 stalks celery, thinly sliced
- 2 cups red seedless grapes, halved

COOKING INSTRUCTIONS

1. Take the honey, poppy seeds, mayo, vinegar, salt and pepper in a bowl and mix it properly.
2. Then chill in the refrigerator for a few minutes.
3. Preheat your oven to 375*F.
4. Arrange the chicken breasts on a baking pan.
5. Cover the pan with foil very well.
6. And Bake it for 25 minutes.
7. Let it cool and then cut it into small cubes.
8. Put the chicken cubes in a large mixing bowl.
9. Add the pecans, celery and grapes in the chicken cubes.
10. Toss with the dressing and then serve it.

ROAST TURKEY WITH APPLES

Yields: 12 servings
Serving Size: 1 portion
Preparation Time: 20 minutes
Cooking Time: 2 hours and 20 minutes
Total Time: 2 hours and 40 minutes

INGREDIENTS

- 5 onions, quarter cut
- Salt and pepper to taste
- 5 apples, peeled, cored and quarter cut
- 2 tbsp. butter, melted
- 2 cloves garlic, chopped
- 1 whole turkey, giblets and neck removed
- ¼ cup fresh sage, chopped

COOKING INSTRUCTIONS

1. First preheat your oven to 475*F.
2. Dry the turkey with paper towels.
3. Brush the outside with butter.
4. Combine garlic, sage, salt and pepper in a bowl and mix it well.
5. Rub the mixture to the outside and also inside of the turkey.
6. Tie the legs of the turkey using (string).
7. Then put the turkey in a roasting pan.
8. Then place it inside the oven and bake for 20 minutes.
9. Place the apple slices and onions around the turkey and roast it for 2 hours more.
10. Leave it sit for 30 minutes before carving (cut into pieces)

CHICKEN BURRITO

Yields: 6 servings
Serving Size: 1 wrap
Preparation Time: 10 minutes
Cooking Time: 10 minutes
Total Time: 20 minutes

INGREDIENTS

- 2 cups roasted chicken meat, shredded
- 6 tbsp. sour cream
- 2 tsp. vegetable oil
- 1 cup salsa
- 3 cups baby spinach leaves, chopped
- 1 onion, diced
- 6 whole wheat tortillas, heated
- 1 cup corn kernels
- 1 ½ cup brown rice, cooked

COOKING INSTRUCTIONS

1. First take vegetable oil in a skillet on medium heat.
2. Sauté the onion into it until it becomes soft.
3. Add the corn kernels into it and keep stirring until it become golden brown.
4. Stir in the rice and chicken.
5. Mix in the sour cream and salsa.
6. Arrange the spinach on top of each tortilla.
7. Ladle the chicken mixture on top.
8. Fold the top part, wrap tightly and secure.
9. Repeat the same recipe with the rest of the tortillas.

ROSEMARY TURKEY BREAST

Yields: 6 servings
Serving Size: 1 turkey breast fillet
Preparation Time: 20 minutes
Cooking Time: 1 hour and 45 minutes
Total Time: 2 hours and 5 minutes

INGREDIENTS

- 5 lb. turkey breast fillet
- 2 tbsp. butter, melted
- 1 ¾ tsp. coarse sea salt
- 1 tbsp. fresh rosemary leaves, chopped
- 2 tbsp. fresh sage leaves, chopped
- 1 tsp. ground black pepper

COOKING INSTRUCTIONS

1. First preheat your oven to 325*F.
2. Then in a bowl take the herbs, salt and pepper and mix it well.
3. Rub the upper part of turkey fillets with butter.
4. Spray the herb mixture all over the turkey.
5. Arrange properly the fillets on a baking pan.
6. Then roast it for 1 hour and 15 minutes.
7. And increase the temperature to 425*F.
8. Roast the turkey for 30 minutes.
9. Leave it cool in refrigerator for 15 minutes.
10. Serve it while warm.

BAKED CHICKEN PARMESAN

Yields: 6 servings
Serving Size: 1 chicken breast fillet
Preparation Time: 15 minutes
Cooking Time: 40 minutes
Total Time: 55 minutes

INGREDIENTS

- 2 tbsp. fresh thyme, chopped
- 1 egg
- 6 chicken breast fillets, boneless and skinless
- ¼ cup low fat milk
- ½ cup Parmesan cheese, grated
- Cooking spray
- ¾ cup panko breadcrumbs
- ¾ tsp. fine sea salt

COOKING INSTRUCTIONS

1. First preheat your oven up to 425*F.
2. Put a wire rack on the top of your baking pan.
3. Coat this with cooking oil spray.
4. Get a mixing bowl and mix the egg and milk properly.
5. In another bowl combine the cheese, breadcrumbs, salt and thyme and mix it well.
6. Dip each of the chicken fillets in the egg mixture and then dredge with the breadcrumb mixture.
7. Then put the breaded chicken pieces on the wire rack.
8. Bake in the oven for 35 - 40 minutes or until it becomes golden brown.

CHICKEN POSOLE

Yields: 8 servings
Serving Size: 1 bowl
Preparation Time: 15 minutes
Cooking Time: 30 minutes
Total Time: 45 minutes

INGREDIENTS

- 1 tbsp. canola oil
- ⅛ tsp. cayenne pepper
- 1 onion, diced
- 2 ½ cups corn kernels
- 2 limes, sliced into wedges
- 5 cups chard leaves and stems, chopped
- 3 tbsp. oregano, chopped
- 5 Poblano peppers, sliced
- 5 ½ cup reduced sodium chicken stock
- ½ tsp. sea salt
- 1 ½ lb. chicken breast (boneless and skinless)
- 5 cloves garlic, minced

COOKING INSTRUCTIONS

1. Pour the canola oil in a soup pot on medium heat.
2. Then add   onion, garlic and peppers in the oil.
3. And cook it for 8 minutes.
4. Add the stock, salt and chicken in the mixture.
5. Then cook it for 20 minutes.
6. Remove pot from heat.
7. Remove the chicken and shred it or chop it on a chopping board very well.
8. Then pour it again to the pot and add the corn, chard and oregano.
9. Season with the cayenne and garnish with the lime wedges before serving.

CHAPTER TEN

VEGAN/VEGETARIAN RECIPES

VEGAN DEVILED "EGGS"

Yields: 12 servings
Serving Size: 1 "egg"
Preparation Time: 15 minutes
Cooking Time: 30 minutes
Total Time: 45 minutes

INGREDIENTS

- ¼ cup silken tofu, drained
- ½ cup vegan mayonnaise
- 12 baby potatoes, sliced in half crosswise
- 2 tsp. extra-virgin olive oil
- 1 tsp. turmeric
- 1 tbsp. Dijon mustard
- ½ tsp. coarse sea salt
- Cooking spray
- ¼ tsp. freshly ground black pepper
- 1 tsp. sweet paprika

COOKING INSTRUCTIONS

1. Preheat your oven up to 350*F.
2. Spray baking pan with cooking spray.
3. Put the potatoes in a large mixing bowl.

4. Then pour the olive oil over the potatoes and toss to blend it well.
5. Lay them on baking pan with the cut-side down.
6. And roast for 30 minutes.
7. Take the potatoes out of the oven and let it cool.
8. Scoop out the middle part of the potatoes.
9. Put this in the food processor along with the rest of the ingredients.
10. Blend it until it becomes smooth.
11. Stuff the potato into halves with this mixture.
12. Chill in the refrigerator for half hour before serving.

TEMPEH AND TOFU DISH

Yields: 4 servings
Serving Size: 1 bowl
Preparation Time: 10 minutes
Cooking Time: 35 minutes
Total Time: 45 minutes

INGREDIENTS

- 2 tbsp. parsley, chopped
- ½ cup tempeh, sliced
- 20 oz. jasmine rice, cooked
- 2 cloves garlic, crushed and minced
- 1 green bell pepper, chopped
- 1 cup celery, chopped
- 1 onion, chopped
- 14.5oz. canned kidney beans
- ½ cup tofu, sliced

COOKING INSTRUCTIONS

1. First cook the tempeh in a skillet for 20 minutes.
2. Then add the onion, garlic, bell pepper and celery. And cook for 5 minutes.
3. Pour this mixture into a soup pot.
4. Add the tofu and beans into it.
5. Then cover the pot.
6. Simmer it for 30 minutes.
7. Serve tempeh mixture with cooked rice and parsley.

SCRAMBLED PEPPERS & MUSHROOMS

Yields: 4 servings
Serving Size: 1 cup
Preparation Time: 15 minutes
Cooking Time: 10 minutes
Total Time: 25 minutes

INGREDIENTS

- 1 tsp. dried basil
- ½ tsp. curry powder
- 1 onion, chopped
- ½ tsp. granulated garlic
- 6 fresh mushrooms, chopped
- ½ green bell pepper, chopped
- Black pepper to taste
- ½ red bell pepper, chopped
- 1 tbsp. reduced sodium tamari
- 1 tsp. vegetable oil
- 1 tbsp. mirin
- 16 oz. firm tofu, drained and mashed

COOKING INSTRUCTIONS

1. Take the vegetable oil into a skillet.
2. Cook the onion, mushroom and bell peppers for 5 minutes in the oil.
3. Mix in the tamari, mirin, tofu, curry powder and garlic.
4. Reduce the heat.
5. And cook for another 5 minutes.
6. Garnish with pepper before serving.

VEGAN FRITTATA WITH ASPARAGUS & TOFU

Yields: 6 servings
Serving Size: 1 slice
Preparation Time: 15 minutes
Cooking Time: 30 minutes
Total Time: 45 minutes

INGREDIENTS

- ½ cup coconut milk
- 14 oz. silken tofu, drained
- Black pepper to taste
- 1 cup leeks, chopped
- ¼ tsp. ground turmeric
- 3 tbsp. nutritional yeast
- ½ cup fresh basil, chopped
- ½ cup asparagus tips
- 1 tbsp. tahini
- 2 tbsp. cornstarch
- 14 oz. firm tofu, drained and crumbled
- ¼ cup Kalamata olives, pitted and chopped

- ½ cup red bell peppers, roasted and chopped

COOKING INSTRUCTIONS

1. Preheat your oven to 400* F.
2. Line an ovenproof skillet with Vellum.
3. Put the coconut milk, silken tofu, tahini, cornstarch, turmeric, yeast and black pepper in a food processor.
4. Blend it until it becomes smooth.
5. Place a skillet over medium heat.
6. Cook the leeks for 5 minutes.
7. Add the asparagus tips, crumbled tofu, olives and red bell peppers into it.
8. Cook for other 5 minutes.
9. Put this and the puréed tofu mixture in a bowl and mix it well.
10. Then add this combination into the ovenproof skillet.
11. Bake it in the oven for 20 minutes.
12. Leave it to cool before slicing.

CAPELLINI & ROASTED VEGGIES

Yields: 4 servings
Serving Size: 1 bowl
Preparation Time: 15 minutes
Cooking Time: 1 hour and 5 minutes
Total Time: 1 hour and 20 minutes

INGREDIENTS

- ½ tsp. arrowroot
- 10 cloves garlic, peeled and sliced in half

- 1 tbsp. balsamic vinegar
- 1 cup red wine
- Black pepper to taste
- 3 tomatoes, cubed
- 1 fennel bulb, cubed
- 2 tsp. olive oil
- ¼ tsp. red chili flakes, crushed
- 8 oz. capellini pasta, cooked according to package directions
- ¼ tsp. dry whole oregano
- 8 oz. cippolini onions, diced

COOKING INSTRUCTIONS

1. First preheat your oven to 375 *F.
2. Put the garlic, onions and olive oil in a baking pan.
3. Toss to blend.
4. Season with the black pepper.
5. And bake for 30 minutes, stirring halfway through.
6. Add the tomatoes, fennel, chili and oregano.
7. Bake for another 15 minutes.
8. Then pour in the vinegar and wine and add the arrowroot.
9. Bake for 25 minutes.
10. Garnish the vegetable mixture by pouring pasta on the top and then serve.

POTATO & MUSHROOM HASH

Yields: 6 servings
Serving Size: 1 cup
Preparation Time: 5 minutes
Cooking Time: 50 minutes
Total Time: 55 minutes

INGREDIENTS

- 4 cloves garlic, crushed and minced
- Chopped parsley for garnish
- 3 purple potatoes, diced
- 1 onion, diced
- 3 large potatoes, diced
- 1 lb. mushrooms, chopped
- 4 fresh sage leaves, sliced thinly

COOKING INSTRUCTIONS

1. Preheat your oven to 375*F.
2. Arrange the potatoes on a baking pan.
3. Roast it for 30 minutes.
4. Place a skillet on medium heat.
5. Sauté the onion and mushrooms for 10 minutes.
6. Then add the roasted potatoes, sage and garlic into it.
7. Cook for addition 10 minutes.
8. Garnish it with the parsley before serving.

VEGAN "HOLLANDAISE" SAUCE

Yields: 2 to 3 servings
Serving Size: 1 tablespoon
Preparation Time: 5 minutes
Cooking Time: 0 minutes
Total Time: 5 minutes

INGREDIENTS

- ¼ tsp. cayenne pepper
- ½ tsp. ground turmeric
- ½ cup warm water
- 2 tsp. Dijon mustard
- 1 tbsp. lemon juice
- ¾ cup organic cashew butter
- 1 tsp. garlic powder
- 1 tsp. lemon zest

COOKING INSTRUCTIONS

1. Take all the ingredients in a blender or food processor.
2. Blend it until becomes smooth.
3. Then serve it with crackers.

TOFU SCRAMBLE

Yields: 4 servings
Serving Size: 1 cup
Preparation Time: 5 minutes
Cooking Time: 8 minutes
Total Time: 13 minutes

INGREDIENTS

- ⅛ tsp. fine sea salt
- ½ yellow bell pepper, quarter-cut
- 3 cloves garlic
- ½ onion, quarter-cut
- 14 oz. firm tofu, drained and crumbled

- 1 tomato, quarter-cut
- 2 cups spinach leaves

COOKING INSTRUCTIONS

1. First add the bell pepper, tomato, spinach, garlic and onion to chopper.
2. Pulse until chopped finely.
3. Then simmer (boil) this mixture in a skillet on medium heat.
4. And add the tofu and season with salt.
5. Cook for 8 minutes.
6. And serve while warm.

VEGETARIAN CHIPOTLE CHILI

Yields: 4 servings
Serving Size: 1 bowl
Preparation Time: 5 minutes
Cooking Time: 35 minutes
Total Time: 40 minutes

INGREDIENTS

- 15 oz. canned kidney beans, rinsed and drained
- ½ cup onion, chopped
- 1 ½ cup bell peppers
- 1 tbsp. chipotle peppers in adobo sauce, chopped
- 1 oz. chili seasoning mix
- 1 cup water
- 2 tbsp. vegetable oil
- 1 tbsp. sour cream
- ½ cup carrot, chopped

- 1 tsp. green onions, chopped
- 15 oz. canned black beans, rinsed and drained
- 28 oz. canned diced tomatoes, undrained
- 2 tbsp. cheddar cheese, grated

COOKING INSTRUCTIONS

1. First pour the vegetable oil into a pot over medium heat.
2. Then cook the onion and carrots into the oil for 3 minutes.
3. Add the bell peppers, chipotles and seasoning and mix it well.
4. And add the water, beans and tomatoes into it.
5. Simmer (boil) for 30 minutes.
6. Then serve it with the cheese, green onions and sour cream.

ALMOND FRENCH TOAST

Yields: 6 servings
Serving Size: 2 bread slices
Preparation Time: 5 minutes
Cooking Time: 5 minutes
Total Time: 10 minutes

INGREDIENTS

- 1 cup unsweetened almond milk
- ¼ tsp. pure almond extract
- ¼ tsp. ground cinnamon
- ¼ cup mashed tofu
- Cooking spray
- 12 slices whole grain bread
- Powdered sugar

- 2 tbsp. almond butter
- 6 tbsp. almonds, toasted and slivered

COOKING INSTRUCTIONS

1. Take the tofu, cinnamon, almond milk, almond extract and almond butter in a blender. Blend it until becomes smooth.
2. Then pour the mixture into a shallow dish.
3. Coat a skillet with cooking oil.
4. Place this on medium heat.
5. Then dip each of the bread slices into the almond milk mixture.
6. Brown it in the skillet.
7. And cook for about 2 minutes.
8. Turn and cook the other side for 2 minutes.
9. Garnish it with the powdered sugar and almonds.

VEGETARIAN BURGER

Yields: 6 servings
Serving Size: 1 round patty and 1 slice cheese
Preparation Time: 30 minutes
Cooking Time: 1 hour and 30 minutes
Total Time: 2 hours

INGREDIENTS

- 1 tsp. sea salt
- Black pepper to taste
- 2 slices bread
- 2 tbsp. extra virgin olive oil, divided
- 1 onion, diced

- 1/4 cup red rice
- 6 slices low fat cheddar cheese
- ½ cup dried porcini mushrooms
- 1 cup hot water
- 2 cloves garlic, crushed and minced
- 1 carrot, diced
- 8 oz. fresh mushrooms, chopped
- 1 tsp. dried thyme

COOKING INSTRUCTIONS

1. First soak the dried mushrooms in hot water for 20 minutes.
2. Satan the liquid and chop the mushrooms on chopping board.
3. Then grind the bread until it turns into fine crumbs.
4. Pour half of the olive oil into a saucepan.
5. Sauté the onion, garlic and carrot in it for 5 minutes.
6. Then add the mushrooms both fresh and dried.
7. Season with the thyme, salt and black pepper.
8. And add the rice and mix it well.
9. Bring to a boil and then simmer for 55 minutes.
10. Mix in the breadcrumbs and transfer the mixture to a bowl.
11. Make 6 round patties from the mixture.
12. Brown patties in the pan for 5 minutes on both sides.
13. Garnish with the cheddar cheese.

ROASTED RATATOUILLE

Yields: 10 servings
Serving Size: 1 cup
Preparation Time: 15 minutes
Cooking Time: 1 hour and 5 minutes

Total Time: 1 hour and 20 minutes

INGREDIENTS

- 1 lb. squash, diced
- ¼ cup olive oil
- 1 lb. eggplant, diced
- ½ lb. yellow onion, diced
- ½ lb. red bell pepper, diced
- 3 tbsp. fresh oregano, chopped
- 3 cloves garlic, crushed and minced
- 3 oz. capers, drained
- ¼ tsp. freshly ground black pepper

- ¼ tsp. fine sea salt
- 1 lb. large tomatoes, diced
- 1 lb. zucchini, diced

COOKING INSTRUCTIONS

1. First preheat your oven to 400*F.
2. Toss the eggplant in salt. Drain in a colander.
3. In a large bowl, mix the tomatoes, oregano, garlic and black pepper.
4. Then in a separate bowl, toss the eggplant, bell pepper, onion, zucchini and squash with olive oil.
5. And put the vegetable mixture in a baking pan.
6. Bake for 45 minutes.
7. Pour the tomato mixture on upper.
8. And bake for another 20 minutes.
9. Add the capers into it and mix before serving.

EGGPLANT VEGAN "BACON

Yields: 8 servings
Serving Size: 3 to 4 slices
Preparation Time: 2 hours 10 minutes
Cooking Time: 1 hour and 30 minutes
Total Time: 3 hours and 40 minutes

INGREDIENTS

- 1 tbsp. olive oil
- 2 tbsp. cider vinegar
- ½ tsp. smoked paprika
- 1 ½ tsp. fine sea salt
- 1 eggplant, sliced lengthwise in quarters
- ¼ cup brown sugar
- 1 tbsp. low sodium tamari
- ¼ cup water
- Cooking spray

COOKING INSTRUCTIONS

1. Slice the eggplant very thinly.
2. Place it in a sifter.
3. Sprinkle with the salt.
4. Wait for 1 hour to get rid of the excess moisture.
5. Rinse and pat dry with paper towels.
6. In a small bowl, blend the water, vinegar, sugar, tamari, oil and paprika very well.
7. Then marinate the eggplant slices in this mixture for 1 hour.
8. After then preheat your oven to 250* F.
9. Grease the baking pan.
10. Arrange the eggplant slices in a single layer.
11. And bake it for 1 hour and a half, or until it becomes crispy.

TEMPEH STROGANOFF

Yields: 4 servings
Serving Size: 1 bowl
Preparation Time: 15 minutes
Cooking Time: 15 minutes
Total Time: 30 minutes

INGREDIENTS

- ½ onion, sliced thinly
- 2 cloves garlic, crushed and minced
- 1 tbsp. vegetable oil
- 2 cups brown rice, cooked
- 2 tbsp. parsley, chopped
- 1 tsp. sesame oil, toasted
- 4 oz. reduced fat vegan sour cream
- 1 tbsp. vegetarian Worcestershire sauce
- 1 large Portobello mushroom, stem removed and sliced
- 1 pack vegetarian gravy mix, prepared according to package directions
- 8 oz. tempeh, cut into strips

COOKING INSTRUCTIONS

1. Pour the vegetable oil into a skillet on medium heat.
2. Then cook the tempeh strips until golden brown on both sides.
3. And remove from the pan and set aside.
4. Cook the onion and garlic in the same pan for 5 minutes.
5. Pour in the sesame oil and Worcestershire sauce.
6. Add the mushrooms and cook until soft.
7. Return the tempeh to the pan.
8. And mix in the prepared gravy mixture.
9. Add the vegan sour cream.
10. Cook until warm.

11. Put rice on the top and garnish with the parsley.

VEGAN BREAD PUDDING

Yields: 8 servings
Serving Size: 1 cup
Preparation Time: 10 minutes
Cooking Time: 1 hour
Total Time: 1 hour and 10 minutes

INGREDIENTS

- ¼ cup fresh chives
- 6 cups whole grain bread cubes
- ⅓ cup flaxseed meal
- 1 lb. silken tofu
- 12 oz. tempeh strips, crumbled
- 1 lb. asparagus, trimmed, sliced and divided
- ¼ tsp. fine sea salt
- Cooking spray
- 3 cups unsweetened almond milk
- ¼ tsp. freshly ground black pepper
- ¼ cup fresh parsley

COOKING INSTRUCTIONS

1. Preheat your oven to 350* F.
2. Coat a casserole dish with cooking spray.
3. In a food processor, add the almond milk, flaxseed meal, tofu, salt and pepper.
4. In a dish, mix the parsley, chives, bread cubes and tempeh.
5. Pour the almond milk mixture onto the bread mixture.

6. Transfer to your casserole and press down gently.
7. Spread a layer of the asparagus on top of it.
8. Then bake it for 50 minutes.

CONCLUSION

In order to live healthy, you have to watch what you eat. If you want to stay free from ailments and all sorts of health conditions, it is a must to eat natural whole foods. Whole food diet help you to achieve this goal by emphasizing whole foods and eliminating foods that have adverse negative effect on your health for 30 days. A diet on Whole foods help you to care about what you put in your body, and focusing your attention on health. With this type of diets, you will also enjoy delicious and satisfying dishes without putting your health at risk.

****

Thanks for reading! If you enjoyed this book or found it useful I'd be very grateful if you'd post a short review on the site you purchased this book from. Your support really does make a difference and I read all the reviews personally so I can get your feedback and make this book even better.

"Thanks again for your support!"